# LIVING WITH HEART DISEASE

# Living with Heart Disease

### BY

**MARIE R. SQUILLACE, M.A.**

**KATHY DELANEY, R.N., B.S.N.**

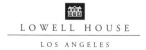

LOWELL HOUSE

LOS ANGELES

CONTEMPORARY BOOKS

CHICAGO

**Library of Congress Cataloging-in-Publication Data**

Squillace, Marie R.
    Living with heart disease / by Marie R. Squillace, Kathy Delaney.
       p.   cm.
    Includes bibliographical references and index.
    ISBN 1–56565–877–9
    1. Heart—Diseases—Popular works.    I. Delaney, Kathy.
II. Title.
RC672.S68   1998
616.1'2—dc21                               97–47284
                                                     CIP

Requests for such permissions should be addressed to:
Lowell House
2020 Avenue of the Stars, Suite 300
Los Angeles, CA 90067

Lowell House books can be purchased at special discounts when ordered in bulk for premiums and special sales.

Publisher: Jack Artenstein
Associate Publisher, Lowell House Adult: Bud Sperry
Director of Publishing Services: Rena Copperman
Managing Editor: Maria Magallanes
Text design: Laurie Young
Illustrations by: Elizabeth Weadon Massari and Susan Spellman

Manufactured in the United States of America
10 9 8 7 6 5 4 3 2 1

Grateful acknowledgment is made to the following contributors:

"Blood Pressure Classifications and Recommendations" is reprinted from the 1993 Report of the Joint National Committee on Detection, Evaluation, and Treatment of High Blood Pressure.

"Ideal Height and Weight Ranges" is reprinted from U.S. Department of Agriculture and the Department of Health and Human Services' Weight Guidelines for Adults, 1995.

"Calculating Body Mass Index" is reprinted from Bray, G. A. and D. S. Gray. "Obesity." *Western Journal of Medicine* (1988) 149:429–441 .

"Eight Guidelines for Discussing Illness with Children" is reprinted with permission by W. M. Sotile. In *Psychosocial Interventions for Cardiopulmonary Patients*, pp. 149–150. Champaign, Ill.: Human Kinetics Publishers, 1996.

"Target Heart Rates" and "How to Evaluate Science News Stories (Steps 1–9)" are reproduced with permission by American Heart Association World Wide Web Site, *Heart and Stroke Guide Section.* Copyright 1996 by the American Heart Association.

"Stress Symptom Checklist" is reprinted with permission by David Hyde, Ph.D., Department of Health Education, University of Maryland.

"Progressive Muscular Relaxation" is reprinted with permission by Glenn R. Schiraldi © 1997 from *Conquer Anxiety, Worry, and Nervous Fatigue: A Guide to Greater Peace*. Ellicott City, Md.: Chevron Publishing, 1997.

"The Air Quality Forecast and Action Guide" is reprinted with permission by the Metropolitan Washington Council of Governments.

"Support Through the Stages of Change," is adapted from "The Role of Social Support in the Modification of Risk Factors for Cardiovascular Disease" by T. L. Amick and J. K. Ockene. In *Social Support and Cardiovascular Disease*, eds. S. A. Shumaker and S. M. Czajkowski, p. 266. New York: Plenum Publishing, 1994. Reprinted with permission.

# Acknowledgments

The authors wish to thank the following individuals for their kindness and support throughout this project:

Peggy McCardle, Ph.D., M.P.H.

Jerrold Greenberg, Ed.D.

Tom Delaney

Tammy White, M.S.W.

Sharon Desmond, Ph.D.

David Hyde, Ph.D.

Glenn Schiraldi, Ph.D.

Teresa Shattuck, M.A.

Karen Olk

Robert Fay

Our colleagues at the INOVA Alexandria Hospital, Alexandria, Virginia

The participants in the INOVA Alexandria Hospital Cardiopulmonary Rehabilitation Program who shared their experiences to make the road easier for others

*To my readers:*
*Knowing what is possible is your new beginning.*

—Marie


*To Tom, Kelly, Ryan, and Katie.*
*Always my source of encouragement, support, and love.*

—Kathy

# Contents

The greatest reward for clinicians who work in a cardiac rehabilitation program is seeing the personal transformation that occurs during the early stages of recovery from heart disease. This transformation occurs not only because our patients begin to feel better physically, but also because they have begun to develop an understanding of the emotional issues that go along with being diagnosed with heart disease. In as little as three to six months, they look back at the accumulation of small successes and realize that they feel better than they have in a long time.

*Living with Heart Disease* takes you on this personal journey. By now, you probably realize that heart disease has many dimensions. When faced with a chronic illness, your relationships, job, financial security, and self-esteem suddenly look much less stable. Fear of sickness and death can cause you to create a level of discomfort that interferes with your recovery. Our goal is to help you peel away the layers. Recovery will involve taking a journey within to better understand what led to the development of heart disease and how you are going to gather the strength and motivation to meet the challenges ahead.

We offer a three-step approach to addressing these issues. To take the mystery out of heart disease, we begin by providing a basic explanation of how your heart works, what can go wrong, and how it can be fixed. The next step is to develop a level of understanding of how you can gain control of your personal lifestyle behaviors that may have led to the development of heart disease. There is a strong focus on managing your risk factors, including physical fitness, nutritional awareness, and stress management. The final step is an exploration of the emotional impact of being diagnosed with a chronic illness. We examine the impact on your relationships with family and friends, the emotional issues of returning to work and to other normal routines, and learning to cope with limitations.

Throughout this book we have drawn on twenty years of combined experience in working with individuals who are recovering from heart disease. We share their challenges, setbacks, and inspirations. There are common threads in their stories, and learning from their successes may make your road easier. We encourage you to participate in a cardiac rehabilitation program in your community during the early stages of your recovery. Your recovery will be guided by clinical specialists, and you can hear and share experiences firsthand with individuals who are meeting the same challenges.

Advances in the treatment of heart disease are ongoing. Each decade has brought new insights and medical breakthroughs. We provide you with an overview of the latest treatment options and guide you in evaluating the latest research. Finally, we provide a comprehensive resource section to assist you in obtaining the most current knowledge about heart disease and its treatment.

All information presented is drawn from current research by leading experts. However, each medical history is unique. Therefore, you should always consult with your personal physician to review your specific recovery plans and discuss concerns.

Our final message comes from *our* hearts: You can do this. By reading this book, you already show the necessary interest and determination. We have seen many people like you succeed.

❧

## CHAPTER ONE

# UNDERSTANDING HEART DISEASE

BEING DIAGNOSED WITH HEART DISEASE CAN BE A FRIGHTENING experience. You may be concerned and have questions about living with heart disease. You may have lost your confidence about how active you can be. You may feel scared or angry. These are all very common and normal reactions.

The good news is that heart disease is treatable. Part of your recovery involves coming to grips with being diagnosed with heart disease and exploring what this means to you. First, realize you are not alone. Approximately 15 million Americans currently live with heart disease. Next, you must look at lifestyle choices. Be assured that with a few changes, you can look forward to a happy and healthy future. Visit a cardiac rehabilitation program and you will see people like yourself who have heart disease and are living active, productive lives.

Consider this period a time of personal transformation, a new beginning. Change can at first be unsettling, but it also can be exciting and freeing. You will see differences both physically and emotionally. Your ultimate goal will be to insure good health and the ability to live life to its fullest. Reading this book will give you the guidance and tools you need to be back in control of your future.

In this chapter we will help you understand how your heart works. First, we will establish the groundwork of how your heart should function, what went wrong, and what you can do to prevent problems in the years to come. Second, we will explore the different types of heart disease, and examine how your doctor makes this diagnosis. Third, we will discuss your options for treatment of heart disease. Finally, we will teach you how to respond to chest pain or angina. Armed with this knowledge, you will develop a more confident attitude and be ready to meet the challenges and rewards ahead.

## YOUR HEART AND HOW IT WORKS

Let's take a journey through your cardiovascular system. The cardiovascular system consists of your heart and an extensive network of blood vessels that transport blood and nutrients throughout your body.

The heart itself is a hollow muscular pump that moves about 2,100 gallons of blood a day throughout the body. The heart is a muscle about the size of your fist. To complete its job, it must pump about seventy times each minute. To visualize this, clench your fist and then open and close it seventy times in a minute. Each time you squeeze your fist closed, imagine blood being forced through your body.

Blood is always being pushed in a forward direction. It moves through four chambers in the heart, the right atrium and ventricle and the left atrium and ventricle (see Figure 1.1). Blood enters the right side of the heart and passes first into the right atrium, then into the right ventricle. From here it is pumped into the lungs to receive oxygen. Blood flows from the lungs into the left atrium, and then into the left ventricle. The left ventricle is the workhorse of the heart because it pumps blood into the rest of the body by way of blood vessels called arteries and veins.

Heart valves separate each chamber to prevent the backflow of blood. They are like one-way doors that allow blood to flow forward into the next chamber. The tricuspid valve separates the right atrium from the right ventricle; the mitral valve separates the left atrium from the left ventricle; the pulmonic valve separates the right ventricle from the pulmonary artery and lungs; and the aortic valve separates the left ventricle from the aorta. The septum is a wall that separates the right and left sides of the heart.

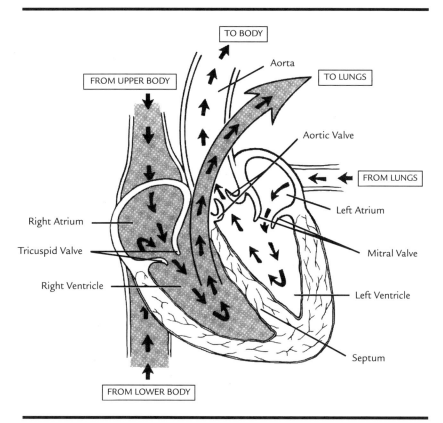

**FIGURE 1.1    Heart Anatomy**
Illustration by Elizabeth Weadon Massari

Just like other muscles, the heart requires its own blood supply to do its work. The blood vessels that feed the heart are called the coronary arteries (see Figure 1.2). The right coronary artery brings blood to the right side and back of the heart. The left coronary artery has two branches: the circumflex and the left anterior descending. These branches carry blood to the septum and left side of the heart.

An electrical system in your heart triggers its pumping action. The sinoatrial node (SA node) in the right atrium is a group of electrical cells that start each beat. The electrical impulse travels from the SA node to the atrioventricular node (AV node) to connect the activity between the atria and ventricles. The bundle branches carry the signal through the ventricles (see Figure 1.3).

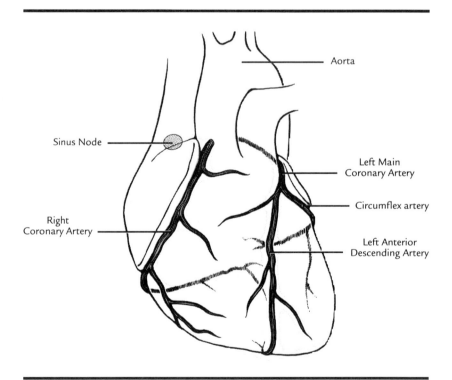

**FIGURE 1.2    Coronary Arteries**
Illustration by Elizabeth Weadon Massari

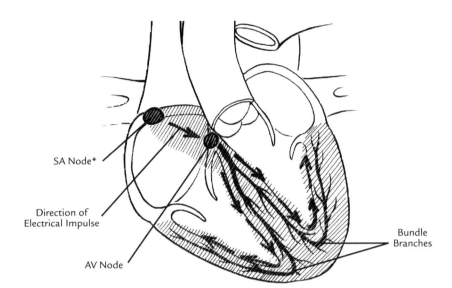

SA Node*

Direction of
Electrical Impulse

AV Node

Bundle
Branches

*The SA node is a group of cells in the heart's upper chamber (atrium). In a normal heartbeat, these cells send an electrical impulse through the AV node (between the heart's upper and lower chambers). The impulse then travels through the bundle branches into the lower chambers to cause a heartbeat.

**FIGURE 1.3    Electrical Conduction**
Illustration by Elizabeth Weadon Massari

Think about the electricity in your house. The electricity is generated from a power plant via power lines to the main electrical circuit in your home, and then to each individual outlet. When the power goes out, you first check to see if it is isolated to one outlet, one room, one level of the house, the whole house, or the whole neighborhood. The same is true with the heart. When there is a problem with the electrical current, you trace the location of the outage: the brain (power plant), the SA node (the main circuit), the AV node (an area circuit), or the bundle branches (the room outlets).

The heart's actions are complex, but we can break them down into understandable steps. Looking at each individual job, you can see how the heart should operate. You will then better understand what happens when something goes wrong.

## UNDERSTANDING HEART DISEASE

It is not uncommon to have more than one heart problem. Heart disease often involves injury to the heart muscle, narrowing of the coronary arteries, and a malfunctioning electrical system, and may also include damage to the heart valves. For example, if you had a heart attack, you may have blockages in your coronary arteries that caused it. You may have an irregular heartbeat due to damage to the heart's electrical circuit, and injury to the heart muscle may weaken your heart's pumping ability. Treatment will be directed at compensating for any injury and preventing future complications.

Once again, visualize the opening and closing of your fist to illustrate your heart's action. Open and close your fist 70 times in one minute to simulate the pumping action of your heart. Now open and close your fist without using two of your fingers. You can see how your pumping ability is limited when only half of your fist is able to open and close. The same is true when the heart muscle is damaged. Now open and close your fist 40 times per minute, and then 140 times per minute. You can see that when there is damage to its electrical system, the heart beats too slow or too fast and, in either case, ineffectively. It cannot keep up with the body's demand for oxygen-rich blood. Treatment is needed to return the heart's function to normal.

### Coronary Artery Disease

As we have seen, the coronary arteries wrap around the top of the heart muscle and provide the heart with a continuous supply of oxygen-rich blood. The inside walls of these arteries are normally smooth and flexible. However, over time these arteries may become clogged and narrowed with fatty deposits called plaque. This narrowing reduces blood flow to the heart muscle, which can cause angina or chest pain.

You experience a heart attack when the narrowed portion of the artery completely closes and cuts off all blood supplying an area of the heart muscle. If an area of the heart muscle does not receive blood flow for longer than fifteen minutes, the heart muscle may be permanently damaged.

## Heart Rhythm Problems

How fast your heart beats and the pattern of the beat are controlled by the electrical system that runs through your heart. When there is a problem with electrical conduction, you may feel palpitations, dizziness, or weakness, and/or you may experience fainting spells. The most common cause of these symptoms is that the heart is not pumping blood effectively. It may be beating too fast, too slow, or too irregularly. There is not enough blood being moved throughout the body.

## Heart Valve Disease

Many people are born with heart valve leakage. As discussed, heart valves act as one-way doors to keep blood flowing in one direction. When there is damage to the heart valves, these valves allow backward blood flow. Your doctor will call this a heart murmur. If there is only a small leak, you may not even know you have this problem, and it may never cause serious difficulties for you. If the leak becomes larger, however, you may begin to experience shortness of breath, fatigue, palpitations, and possibly chest pain.

## Heart Failure

The three most common causes of heart failure are heart attack, high blood pressure, and cardiomyopathy, a disease of the heart muscle. The heart muscle can be weakened as a result of a heart attack that damages a portion of it. Long-term high blood pressure can cause the heart to enlarge due to the extra work involved in pumping the blood. Cardiomyopathy can cause your entire heart muscle to become enlarged and inefficient. Whatever the cause, the end result is the same. The damaged heart pumps blood with inadequate force. This causes blood to back up into the lungs and blood vessels. You may experience shortness of breath, swelling of your ankles and feet, fatigue, cough, and weight gain.

## DIAGNOSIS OF HEART DISEASE

Your doctor will begin your evaluation by reviewing your symptoms and medical history and performing a medical examination. You can help by anticipating questions and giving clear answers. Questions you can expect to be asked include the following:

- What are the symptoms you are experiencing (a symptom describes how you feel at a particular time)? Do you feel sick? Do you have pain? Where is the pain? Describe the pain. When you experience these symptoms do you feel hot or cold? Do you feel sick to your stomach? Are you short of breath? Can you think clearly? Do you feel tired? Do you notice any heart palpitations (irregular heartbeats)?
- What are you doing when you experience the symptoms? Do you notice any pattern to what triggers the symptoms? At what time of day do the symptoms occur, and how long do they last?
- What makes the symptoms go away? How long does it take for the symptoms to go away?
- What is your family medical history? Is there a history of heart disease, diabetes, cancer, or lung disease in your family?
- Have you been under any unusual stress (job, relationships, financial, etc.)?

- What type of diet do you follow (high fat, low fat, frequent fast-food meals, food variety, etc.)?

In addition to gathering this information, your doctor will perform a complete physical examination. This exam evaluates your heart rate, breathing rate, blood pressure, height and weight, heart sounds, lung sounds, reflexes, mental alertness, and any symptoms that may suggest fluid retention such as ankle swelling. A routine blood analysis will also be part of this assessment. Your doctor uses this initial evaluation to determine what additional testing needs to be done. Testing may include electrocardiogram, stress test, X ray, echocardiogram, cardiac catheterization, Holter monitor, and electrophysiology studies.

## Electrocardiogram (EKG)

An electrocardiogram measures the electrical activity of your heart, detected by electrodes attached to your chest. This information is displayed on a screen and usually printed out, so that your doctor can evaluate your heart rate and heart rhythm. Different waves represent electrical activity in different areas of your heart. An electrocardiogram can provide evidence of earlier heart attacks. Changes in wave forms on the EKG may alert your doctor to possible problems with your heart that require more detailed evaluation.

## Stress Testing

Stress testing is like an EKG that shows your heart's response to exercise. The test is usually performed while you are walking on a treadmill or pedaling a stationary bike. If you are unable to exercise, your heart rate can also be artificially stimulated with medication. Stress testing evaluates your heart at work. The narrowing of blood vessels becomes more of a problem when the heart is working hard. If there is an area of your heart not receiving enough oxygen during exercise, you may experience chest pain or shortness of breath, and the EKG may show changes that could indicate a problem with one of the arteries of your heart.

Another type of stress test is a thallium treadmill test. This is a more detailed test because it shows blood flow through the heart muscle both at rest and during exercise by using a radioactive substance called thallium. For this test, the doctor will ask you to walk on a treadmill and then give you an injection of the radioisotope thallium. Scanning is done at peak exercise and again hours later at rest. If no thallium shows up on the images, it may indicate an area of the heart muscle that is not receiving proper blood supply. Absence of blood flow at rest and with exercise may indicate permanent damage to the heart muscle from a previous heart attack. If blood flow is absent with exercise but returns after rest, this may indicate a narrowing of a coronary artery that puts a part of the heart muscle in danger during exercise.

Stress testing helps to identify whether you have coronary artery disease and whether you are at risk for future complications. It can also help determine the effectiveness of certain medications, and identifies safe limits for you for your daily activities and exercise routines. Further testing may be necessary if abnormal results are present.

## X Rays

X rays determine if there are any lung conditions present that may be causing symptoms, such as pneumonia. They also show evidence of heart enlargement or heart failure.

## Echocardiogram

An echocardiogram is an ultrasound study that provides two-dimensional imaging of your heart. It helps to analyze the pumping action of the heart by indicating blood flow and movement of the heart muscle. It can also show the motion of your valves, and help your doctor determine if the valves are opening and closing properly. The size and thickness of the heart muscle and chambers also can be evaluated.

## Cardiac Catheterization

Cardiac catheterization, also known as a coronary angiogram, refers to X ray visualization of heart anatomy using contrast dye. It involves inserting a catheter (a long, thin, flexible tube) into an artery in your groin that is then guided into your heart. Special X rays are used to guide the catheter and visualize the heart. Dye is injected from the catheter into the coronary arteries to see if you have any narrowing or blockages of your arteries. The doctor also evaluates the pumping action of your heart and whether there are any problems with your heart valves. The cardiac catheterization provides information about your individual anatomy for the doctor as well.

**DIAGNOSIS:**
**CORONARY ARTERY DISEASE AND HEART FAILURE**

The following assessment and procedures may be part of your evaluation for coronary artery disease and heart failure.

- Medical history
- Physical assessment
- Blood analysis
- X ray
- Electrocardiogram
- Echocardiogram
- Stress test
- Cardiac catheterization

## EXPLORING THE CAUSE OF
## AN IRREGULAR HEART RHYTHM

If you are being evaluated for an irregular heart rhythm, your evaluation may include all of the testing already described such as blood analysis, X ray, electrocardiogram, echocardiogram, stress test, and cardiac catheterization. Additionally, there are special tests available that help your doctor evaluate what is triggering the abnormal heart rhythm. These include Holter monitoring and electrophysiology studies.

### Holter Monitoring

Holter monitoring is used to look for abnormalities of your heart rhythm. Electrodes are attached to your chest and your heart rhythm is recorded for twenty-four hours using a cassette recorder worn around your waist. You may be asked to keep a written record of your activities during this time. All of this information helps to determine at what points you have abnormal heart rhythms. Changes in the electrocardiogram may also indicate areas of the heart that are not receiving enough oxygen.

### Electrophysiology Studies

Electrophysiology studies may be recommended when your doctor suspects that you have a serious heart rhythm irregularity that needs further evaluation. As in a cardiac catheterization, a catheter is inserted into an artery, usually through the groin, and is guided into your heart. The catheter electrodes stimulate different areas of the electrical system to map the electrical conduction of your heart. In this way, your doctor can identify the area of the heart which is triggering the irregular heart rhythm. Once the doctor has this information, he/she will try various medications to see which one works best for you to prevent this problem from occurring.

**DIAGNOSIS:**

**IRREGULAR HEART RHYTHM**

The following assessment and procedures may be completed during your evaluation for an irregular heart rhythm.

- Medical history
- Physical assessment
- Blood analysis
- Electrocardiogram
- Echocardiogram
- Stress test
- Cardiac catheterization
- Holter monitoring
- Electrophysiology studies

## EXPLORING YOUR OPTIONS: TREATMENT OF HEART DISEASE

You can expect that treatment for your heart condition will be approached in multiple ways that will include risk factor management, medication, and one or more procedures such as angioplasty, stent placement, atherectomy, or surgery for coronary artery disease; balloon valvuloplasty or valve replacement surgery for heart valve disease; or pacemaker, cardioversion, catheter ablation, and/or implanted cardioversion defibrillator for irregular heart rhythms. A heart transplant may be considered when heart failure is no longer responding to medication. As with all medical practice, there is judgment involved in determining the best course of treatment for you. It is important that you be actively involved in this process. Your doctor should encourage questions and take time to be sure that you understand all treatment options.

## Risk Factor Management

The first step in managing your heart disease is a decision only you can make. Are you willing to take control of the risk factors that may have led to the development of heart disease? Think of when you have a clogged kitchen sink. You do what is necessary to unclog the drain and then find out what you need to do to prevent it from happening again. Now ask yourself what led to blockages developing in your coronary arteries, and what you can do to prevent this from happening in the future. High cholesterol, high blood pressure, smoking, obesity, inactivity, diabetes, and stress are the major risk factors that contribute to the development of heart disease. Your challenge is to follow a low-fat, low-cholesterol diet, maintain your ideal body weight, develop stress management skills, exercise, and stop smoking if you currently smoke. Chapter 2 provides a detailed description of all the risk factors and presents strategies to reduce your chances of future complications.

## Medication

Medications may be used alone or in combination with other treatments. They are directed at controlling your symptoms and preventing future complications. Medications may be prescribed to control high blood pressure, prevent angina, control your heart rhythm, prevent clots from forming, or control high cholesterol levels. Although recommended doses are prescribed based on available research, how your body responds to a medication can be very individualized. It is not uncommon for your doctor to have to experiment to find the right doses of medication for you. It can sometimes take several adjustments to come up with the right combination of medicines at the correct doses to control your symptoms and prevent complications, so be patient and don't give up hope.

## Treatment Options: Coronary Artery Disease

In addition to lifestyle changes and medication, treatment for coronary artery disease will be aimed at improving blood flow through the narrowed arteries by reducing plaque buildup, or providing an alternate route for blood flow by bypassing the blockages. Current options include percutaneous transluminal coronary angioplasty (PTCA), stent placement, atherectomy, and heart surgery.

### *Angioplasty*

Angioplasty (also known as PTCA or percutaneous transluminal coronary angioplasty) is a nonsurgical procedure typically used for treatment of one or two blockages of the coronary arteries. During angioplasty, a balloon-tipped catheter is fed through an artery (usually the femoral artery in the groin) into the coronary artery, guided by X ray. At the site of the blockage the balloon is inflated, forcing the plaque to be compressed against the artery wall, and the blockage is reduced, resulting in improved blood flow through the artery (see Figure 1.4). Your doctor will evaluate the number of blockages, their size and distribution, and the size of the artery when determining if this is a good option for you. For multiple blockages or more complex blockages, bypass surgery may be a better treatment option.

The advantage of PTCA is that you are kept awake during the procedure and can look forward to a very quick recovery. However, one-third of all angioplasties close within the first six months. This will require a follow-up procedure, such as a repeat angioplasty, stent placement, or bypass surgery to open this artery again.

### *Stent*

A coronary stent is a small metal coil that is placed in a coronary artery to keep it open (see Figure 1.5). The procedure is similar to heart catheterization or angioplasty. Under X ray guidance, a catheter is inserted through the artery in the groin and guided to the coronary artery. With stent placement, the tip of the catheter is

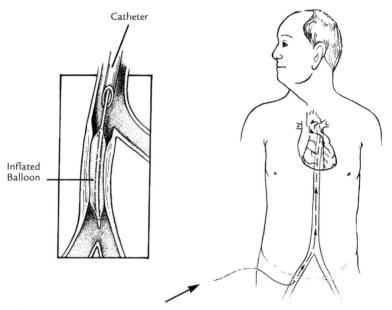

A balloon catheter is inserted through the aorta into the blocked artery

**FIGURE 1.4    Angioplasty**
Illustration by Elizabeth Weadon Massari

mounted with the stent. After the angioplasty is completed, the stent is put in place and pressed against the inner wall of the coronary artery at the site of the blockage. The stent remains in place to keep the artery open. Research has shown that stent placement may improve the success rate of angioplasty.

### *Atherectomy*

Atherectomy is a procedure involving the insertion of a catheter through the artery in the groin and threading it to the blockage in the coronary artery in a procedure similar to cardiac catheterization and angioplasty (see Figure 1.6). With this procedure, however, the catheter contains a rotating disk that shaves off plaque and collects it in a storage chamber for removal from the body. Compared to

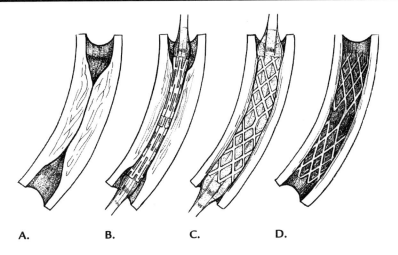

A. Coronary arterial blockage pre-treatment

B. Stent in place before expansion over balloon catherter

C. Expanded stent over balloon catheter

D. Expanded stent in place after removal of balloon catheter

**FIGURE 1.5    Stent**
Illustration by Elizabeth Weadon Massari

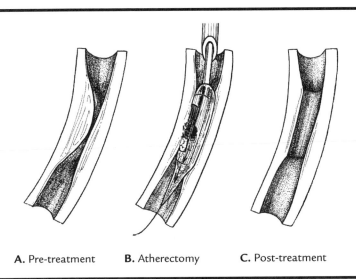

**A.** Pre-treatment    **B.** Atherectomy    **C.** Post-treatment

**FIGURE 1.6    Atherectomy**
Illustration by Elizabeth Weadon Massari

angioplasty or stent placement, where the plaque is compressed against the artery, during atherectomy the plaque is actually removed. The result is a wider opening in the artery.

### *Heart Surgery*

You will be considered for coronary artery bypass graft (CABG) surgery if you have multiple blockages of the coronary arteries, or if the blockages are not accessible by catheter for an angioplasty, stent, or atherectomy. Bypass surgery provides an alternative pathway for blood flow to the heart, bypassing a blocked coronary artery (see Figure 1.7). Several blockages can be bypassed during the same surgery. A leg vein or internal mammary artery in the chest is used to provide this alternate passage. This is a surgical procedure that involves opening the chest wall and possibly the leg (to remove a leg vein to be used for the bypass graft). It requires general anesthesia, typically hospitalization for four to seven days, and a recovery period of six to eight weeks. This surgery has been very successful in helping people feel well again. Ninety percent of patients experience relief of symptoms through bypass surgery. The long-term success of the surgery depends on how well you take care of yourself after surgery. You can expect the bypass grafts to remain open for an average of about ten years if you live a healthy lifestyle that includes controlling all of your risk factors (see chapter 2).

Newly introduced in the arena of heart operations is minimally invasive heart surgery. This surgery involves a smaller incision, faster recovery, and less pain. It is currently being used for single or double artery bypass surgery and aortic and mitral valve repair. It replaces the traditional large incision and may not require use of the heart-lung machine (used while the heart is stopped during the traditional bypass surgery). When the heart-lung machine is not used, the challenge to the surgeon is to develop skill at sewing on a beating heart. Not everyone is eligible for this surgery; it depends on the number and location of the blockages.

Imagine a rock slide in the mountains. Initial road reconstruction will depend on the extent of damage to area roads. The questions will be: Can the rocks be removed or pushed to the side, or is the distribution of the rocks so extensive that it would be better just to bypass the road with a new highway? This is what your doctors must consider when they determine what the best course of treatment will be for you: angioplasty, atherectomy, or heart surgery.

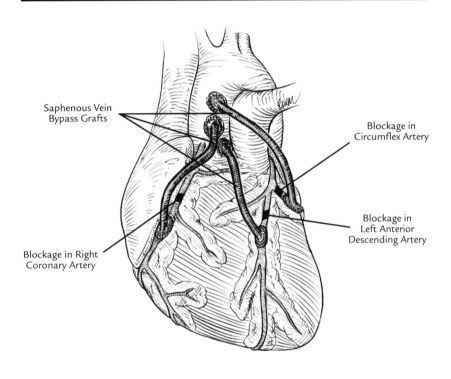

**FIGURE 1.7   Heart Surgery**
Illustration by Elizabeth Weadon Massari

**TREATMENT OPTIONS:**
**CORONARY ARTERY DISEASE**

- Medication
- Risk factor management
- Percutaneous transluminal coronary angioplasty (PTCA)
- Stent
- Atherectomy
- Heart surgery

## HEART VALVE DISEASE

Remember that heart valves act as one-way doors to keep blood moving forward through the heart. Minor irregularities of the heart valves cause minor backward flow of blood and may go unnoticed throughout your life. Heart valve disease becomes more significant when you develop symptoms: shortness of breath, an irregular heart rhythm, dizziness, fatigue, and possibly chest pain. In addition to medication, options for treatment of heart valve disease include heart valve replacement surgery and balloon valvuloplasty.

A word of caution. People with damaged heart valves often are susceptible to endocarditis. Endocarditis is an inflammation of the membranes inside your heart and heart valves. This inflammation is caused by bacteria commonly found in the mouth and respiratory tract. During dental procedures and surgery, these bacteria may enter your bloodstream; they commonly settle on damaged heart valves. To prevent this from occurring, your doctor may prescribe an antibiotic before dental work or surgery.

## Heart Valve Replacement Surgery

Surgery is required for heart valve disease when the valve becomes so stiff or damaged, or the symptoms become so severe, that your quality of life is becoming seriously compromised. During surgery the damaged heart valve can be reconstructed, or it can be replaced with an artificial valve or a valve from a pig's heart.

## Balloon Valvuloplasty

A procedure similar to angioplasty called balloon valvuloplasty can be used to treat heart valves that stick together because of damage to the valve. During this procedure, a balloon catheter is inserted and inflated at the site of the injured valve to enlarge the opening and restore normal functioning of the heart valve.

**TREATMENT OPTIONS:**
**HEART VALVE DISEASE**
- Medication
- Heart valve replacement surgery
- Balloon valvuloplasty

## IRREGULAR HEART RHYTHMS

When medication does not control an irregular heart rhythm, other options are to interrupt the rhythm and allow the normal electrical circuitry to regain control; to implant a device that artificially paces the heart at a normal rate and rhythm; or to remove or destroy the electrical cells that are causing the irregular rhythm. These options include pacemakers, cardioversion, implantable cardioverter defibrillator (ICD), catheter ablation, or surgery.

## Pacemaker

A pacemaker is a device that is put into your body to help regulate your heart rhythm. When you have a problem with your body's electrical system, your heart may beat too slow or too fast. The pacemaker has a pulse generator that contains a battery and electronic circuit and pacing wires attached to the heart that carry the impulse from the pulse generator to the heart muscle. If the generator senses that the heart rate is too slow, then an electrical signal is triggered to make the heart beat.

## Cardioversion

Cardioversion involves delivery of an electric shock to the heart through the chest wall to restore a normal heart rhythm. The electric shock causes all the electrical activity in the heart to stop momentarily. This allows the normal electrical conduction circuitry to regain control and pace the heart normally again. Cardioversion is usually done as a scheduled procedure in the hospital for treatment of a stable heart rhythm irregularity. Defibrillation is an electric shock delivered in an emergency situation due to a life-threatening irregular heart rhythm.

## Implantable Cardioverter Defibrillator (ICD)

An ICD is a device that is implanted inside the body and is ready to deliver an electric shock to the heart when needed. An ICD is necessary if you experience life-threatening rapid heart rhythm (tachycardia) that cannot consistently be prevented with medication or surgery. Examples of these rhythms are ventricular tachycardia and ventricular fibrillation. These rhythms are life threatening because your heart beats too quickly, which prevents it from filling adequately with blood between beats. In this situation, insufficient blood reaches your brain and other vital body organs. Your heart-pumping action can become so erratic that it stops pumping blood altogether, resulting in cardiac arrest.

The first-line treatment for these types of arrhythmias is defibrillation, which provides an electric shock to the heart to restore it to its normal heart rhythm. The ICD provides ongoing monitoring of your heart rhythm and can save your life by providing an electric shock to the heart and bringing a dangerously fast heart rhythm under control. Similar to a pacemaker, the ICD is implanted inside your body and works automatically. It contains a pulse generator with a battery and electronic circuitry, and lead wires which connect the pulse generator to your heart. Patches at the end of the lead wires are attached to your heart to sense the heart rhythm and deliver the electric shocks as needed.

## Catheter Ablation

Catheter ablation is a procedure that destroys the area of the heart's electrical circuit that is triggering an abnormal heart rhythm. During this procedure, your doctor guides a catheter to the trouble spot. Radiofrequency energy passes through the catheter. The tip of the catheter heats up and destroys the exact area of the heart that is causing the irregular heart rhythm.

## Surgery

In rare instances, your doctor may perform surgery to cut or remove abnormal electrical pathways. This surgery has largely been replaced with other interventions, including catheter ablation.

## HEART FAILURE

As we have discussed, heart failure has many different causes. It may be caused by damage to the heart muscle after a heart attack. Long-term uncontrolled high blood pressure can cause heart enlargement

**TREATMENT OPTIONS:**
**IRREGULAR HEART RHYTHMS**

- Medication
- Pacemaker
- Cardioversion
- Implantable cardioverter defibrillator (ICD)
- Catheter ablation
- Surgery

and a weakened heart muscle. Cardiomyopathy, a disease of the heart muscle, can cause your entire heart to become enlarged. The damaged heart pumps blood with inadequate force. This causes blood to back up into the lungs and tissues, resulting in shortness of breath, swelling of the ankles, fatigue, cough, and weight gain. In all of these situations, the pumping action of the heart is weakened. Treatment of heart failure focuses on treating its cause, as well as the use of medications that decrease the work of the heart. Four common types of medication used to treat heart failure include ACE inhibitors and vasodilators to open up your arteries to make it easier for your heart to pump blood; digitalis to make your heart beat stronger; and diuretics or "water pills" to make your kidneys produce more urine so that fluid does not collect in your lungs, ankles, feet, and abdomen.

You will also be taught to make lifestyle adjustments that decrease the heart's workload, including balancing periods of activity with rest periods, maintaining your ideal body weight, and monitoring fluid and sodium intake to prevent fluid buildup causing ankle swelling and lung congestion. In rare instances, heart transplantation will be considered when your heart no longer responds to medication.

## Heart Transplantation

Heart transplantation may be considered when the heart becomes so weak that long-term survival is limited and your quality of life is severely compromised. This is the last step in the treatment of heart failure caused by damage to the heart muscle.

Unfortunately, there is a shortage of donor hearts available for transplantation. Being accepted as a transplant candidate involves rigorous screening. You must show no signs of infection, other organ systems must be healthy, and you must be motivated to comply with a strict follow-up care regimen that includes doctors' appointments, medication that will help to prevent rejection of your new heart, and rejection testing.

**TREATMENT OPTIONS:**
**HEART FAILURE**

- Medication
- Diet
- Balancing activity and rest periods
- Heart transplant

## ANGINA: A CALL TO ACTION

Angina is the most misunderstood symptom of heart disease. When you experience angina, you may become frightened and uncertain about what action to take. This section will help you understand what angina is, and how to treat it. Think about other chronic illnesses. If you have asthma and begin wheezing, you take the medication your doctor prescribed to relieve the wheezing. If you have a stomach ulcer and develop a stomachache you take the antacid your doctor prescribed. The symptom of wheezing or a stomachache does not necessarily mean something more serious is about to happen. It is a symptom of the disease. You treat the symptom with the medication the doctor prescribed for you. If the usual treatment doesn't work, then you call the doctor. Angina is no different—if you have angina you need to treat it immediately.

Angina pectoris is the medical term for chest pain: "angina" means pain, and "pectoris" means chest. You experience angina when an area of your heart muscle is not receiving enough oxygen. Angina is experienced in differing ways from person to person. Angina is not just chest pain. It can be described as chest tightness, pressure, heaviness, squeezing, burning, aching, pain, fullness, indigestion, or numbness. The discomfort may be located in or spread from the mid or left chest to the neck, jaw, upper back, shoulders, or arms. Other symptoms may include shortness of breath, weakness, nausea, or dizziness.

The increased demand for oxygen that triggers angina may be caused by strenuous exercise, emotional stress, lifting a heavy object, eating a large meal, or environmental conditions such as extreme heat or cold or high altitude. Just as the calf muscles in your leg may become painful from inadequate blood supply if you overexercise, your heart muscle signals discomfort when it is not receiving an adequate oxygen supply.

There are three types of angina—stable, unstable, and variant or Prinzmetal's angina. Your doctor will complete a thorough medical evaluation to determine the cause of your angina. As we discussed, this may include stress testing, a heart catheterization, and/or an echocardiogram. It is during this evaluation that your doctor will determine if the angina you are experiencing is stable. Stable angina means that you are not at immediate risk of further or new injury to your heart muscle. Your symptoms can be controlled with medication and lifestyle adjustments. When you experience stable angina, it usually resolves quickly with rest and possibly nitroglycerin tablets.

Unstable angina is chest pain that can be present at rest or with exercise. It may be newly present in situations that in the past have not triggered an angina episode. It may last longer and/or the usual treatment of rest and nitroglycerin may not work. This is a more serious form of angina because it may signal the development of a new blockage or that your current medication is no longer providing protection to the heart. Unstable angina requires immediate medical attention.

A third type of angina is called variant angina or Prinzmetal's angina. This type of angina is caused by a spasm of the coronary artery which blocks the blood supply to the heart muscle. It can occur at rest as well as during periods of increased demand such as exertion or emotional stress. Although the cause of the angina is spasm (rather than blockage), it still can cause a heart attack. Treatment includes medication to prevent spasm from occurring and nitroglycerin to relax the vessels at the time the episode occurs.

## Angina Triggers

If you have angina, your first goal will be to develop a lifestyle that prevents angina from occurring the majority of the time. Keeping in mind the four E's (exertion, emotion, eating, and environment) will remind you of the most common angina triggers.

### Exertion

Overworking or overexercising can be an angina trigger. Pacing yourself through daily work responsibilities will help you to prevent the onset of angina. Exercising within your target heart rate range will usually prevent angina from occurring with exercise (see chapter 4).

### Emotion

Various emotional states will cause your heart to work harder than it normally needs to while at rest. Practicing the stress management strategies in chapter 6 will help you to control your emotional responses to a variety of emotional states.

### Eating

Eating a large, rich meal requires an increased blood supply to the stomach for digestion. This increases the workload of the heart, which may trigger angina. You should eat three meals a day following the portion sizes and food variety provided by the food pyramid guidelines presented in chapter 5.

### Environment

The body works very hard to maintain a normal body temperature. Exercise in extreme hot or cold temperatures makes your heart work even harder. In addition, high altitudes, humidity, high winds, and polluted air can all trigger angina. (See chapter 7 for weather guidelines.)

## Treatment for Angina

Nitroglycerin is the medication most commonly used for the treatment of angina. Don't hesitate to use it when you are experiencing angina. Remember, you are using nitroglycerin just like the individual with asthma uses an inhaler to control wheezing, or the individual with an ulcer takes an antacid tablet to control stomach pain. Nitroglycerin works by relaxing the blood vessels so that blood flow to the affected area of the heart muscle is restored. It also lowers blood pressure and redistributes blood volume throughout the body. This eases the workload of the heart and should relieve the angina.

When angina occurs, follow these important steps:

1. Slow down and stop what you are doing. Sit down and rest for five minutes.
2. If the angina is still present after five minutes, place one nitroglycerin tablet under your tongue and let it dissolve. Do not chew or swallow the tablet.
3. Continue to take one tablet every five minutes for a total of three tablets if the discomfort is not relieved.

4. If you have taken three nitroglycerin tablets and you still have discomfort, call your local emergency medical system. Do not drive yourself to the hospital.

### *The Many Faces of Nitroglycerin*

Nitroglycerin is usually prescribed by your doctor to treat angina. Nitroglycerin comes in many forms and serves different purposes. Sublingual nitroglycerin is dissolved under the tongue during an angina attack. Its effects should occur within five minutes. Nitroglycerin swallowable tablets and patches or paste prevent the onset of angina by relaxing the coronary arteries and decreasing the workload of the heart. Table 1.1 will help you to see the differences in the various forms of nitroglycerin.

Your doctor may have prescribed other medication for the long-term management of angina. This includes calcium channel blockers and beta blockers. The goal of all medication is to prevent angina from occurring by reducing the work of the heart and to keep you feeling great!

**TABLE 1.1    The Various Forms of Nitroglycerin**

| | USE | HOW SUPPLIED | ONSET OF ACTION | LASTS | DIRECTIONS |
|---|---|---|---|---|---|
| **Nitrostat™** | Relieve angina attack. | Sublingual tablet. Place under tongue to dissolve. | 1–3 minutes | 30 minutes | Take 1 tablet every 5 minutes for a maximum of 3 tablets or until angina relieved. If angina is not relieved after 3 tablets, call emergency medical system. |
| **Nitrolingual™** | Relieve angina attack. | Spray. 1-2 sprays under tongue at onset of angina. | 2 minutes | 30–60 minutes | Take 1-2 sprays every 5 minutes for a maximum of 3 doses or until angina is relieved. If angina is not relieved after 3 doses, call emergency medical system. |
| **Nitrol™, Nitro-Bid Paste™** | Prevent angina attacks. | Ointment or patch. Apply on hairless area of skin. Rotate sites. | 30 minutes | Varies: 12–24 hours | Apply as directed by your physician. May require removal at night to avoid developing tolerance. |

| | | | | | |
|---|---|---|---|---|---|
| **Nitro-Bid**™ | Prevent angina attacks. | Swallowable tablets. | 15–30 minutes | 3–8 hours | Use as directed to prevent angina attacks. |
| **Isosorbide Dinitrate**™, **Isordil**™ | Prevent angina attacks. | Swallowable tablets. | 15–30 minutes | 4–6 hours | |
| **Isosorbide Dinitrate**™, **Isordil**™ | Relieve angina attack. | Sublingual tablet. Place under tongue to dissolve. | 2–5 minutes | 1–4 hours | Take 1 tablet every 5 minutes for a maximum of 3 tablets or until angina relieved. If angina is not relieved after 3 tablets, call emergency medical system. |

**BEST FRIENDS:**
**YOU AND NITROGLYCERIN**

- Carry tablets with you at all times in an outside pocket or purse.
- Keep tablets in their own brown bottle (they are light sensitive).
- Do not put other pills in the bottle with the nitroglycerin.
- Store in a cool, dry place.
- Obtain a new stock bottle every six months to ensure freshness.
- A nitroglycerin tablet should cause a tingling or burning sensation under your tongue. If it does not, it may no longer be fresh or effective.
- Headache is a common side effect. Your doctor may suggest taking acetaminophen to relieve the headache.

## PUTTING IT ALL TOGETHER

Sifting through this information and understanding how your heart works and what went wrong will help you to be a more active participant in your health care. You will do better during your recovery, too.

You are a survivor; you have been given a second chance. The upcoming chapters will teach you how to make the most of this second chance. Those who have already met the challenges of making the necessary lifestyle changes to control their heart disease will tell you that they feel better than they have ever felt in their lives. It's time to begin goal setting.

## A NOTE TO FAMILY AND FRIENDS

This chapter is filled with details about your heart and how it works. It is intended to make you better informed about the heart's functioning and how to recognize when something isn't right. Health care professionals spend their entire careers learning the intricacies of how the heart works and how to treat heart disease. This is not your responsibility. Your responsibility is to provide emotional support, work with your loved one in managing cardiac risk factors, and learn enough about the symptoms of heart disease to be able to identify when a problem is developing. Call the doctor if the following symptoms develop:

- Chest pain (angina). *Chest pain that is unrelieved with three nitroglycerin tablets may be a warning sign of a heart attack. Call 911 for immediate treatment in an emergency room. A delay in treatment may result in further damage to the heart muscle.*
- New shortness of breath at rest or with activity
- Irregular heartbeat
- Unexplained fatigue
- New cough
- Weight gain greater than 2 pounds in one week
- New swelling of the feet or ankles
- Fever
- Nausea
- Difficulty sleeping

## CHAPTER TWO

# CALCULATING YOUR RISKS

LIFE IS FULL OF RISKS. DECISIONS ABOUT CAREER, MARRIAGE, AND financial ventures all involve weighing options and selecting what you believe will lead to the best outcome. This is what managing cardiac risk factors is about. Risk factors are lifestyle behaviors that increase your risk for heart disease. The odds are in your favor that if you make the decision to control your risk factors, you will prevent or limit future health problems. Taking action will give you the satisfaction of knowing that you are doing everything within your ability to ensure a healthy outcome.

This chapter will present the how, what, when, and why you need to manage your risk factors. It is based on scientific research that began with the Framingham Heart Study in 1948. This and other studies have tracked populations of individuals to identify what traits put them at a higher risk for heart disease. Common to the majority of these studies are the following controllable risk factors: high cholesterol, high blood pressure, smoking, diabetes, inactivity, obesity, and stress. Risk factors that cannot be controlled are age, gender, and family history.

The first step in controlling risk factors is to take a personal inventory of those you have that make you susceptible to heart disease.

1. Do you smoke?
2. Do you have elevated total and/or LDL cholesterol or triglyceride levels, or low HDL cholesterol?
3. Do you have elevated blood pressure?
4. Are you physically inactive?
5. Do you have diabetes?
6. Are you under stress that you have difficulty controlling?
7. Are you male or a postmenopausal female?
8. Are you older than age fifty-five?
9. Do you have a family history of heart disease that presented before age fifty-five in men or age sixty-five in women?

Look at those questions 1 to 6 to which you answered yes. These are the risk factors that you need to address. Turn to the sections in this chapter that discuss these risks in greater detail. Gender, family history, and age are risks that you cannot control. However, you can counter balance these risks by controlling all other factors.

Your successful recovery is based on your active involvement in managing your risk factors. Making recommended lifestyle changes will strengthen your heart and help you to maintain a positive outlook for the future.

## CALCULATING THE RISK OF HIGH CHOLESTEROL AND HEART DISEASE

When we think about heart disease, high cholesterol levels are a topic that comes to almost everyone's minds. Too much cholesterol in the blood can cause our arteries to clog up. Frequently we can

**A NOTE TO FAMILY AND FRIENDS**

Your family member or friend is being asked to make lifestyle changes and break habits that took a lifetime to develop. Be patient. Accept small steps forward. Take the risk factor inventory yourself. If your lifestyle habits put you at risk, change with him or her. Your support is essential.

Be aware of your loved one's emotional state. Depression is common when someone is initially diagnosed with heart disease. Symptoms may include social withdrawal, diminished appetite, sleeplessness, lack of energy, inability to make decisions, and tearfulness. If symptoms such as these continue for prolonged periods, it is important to discuss them with the doctor. Untreated depression can delay recovery.

attribute high cholesterol to poor eating habits, such as too many fast-food meals, an addiction to potato chips, or an ice cream obsession. All of this is true, but cholesterol is more complex than this. Abnormal cholesterol levels can be the result not only of poor diet, but also an inactive lifestyle, or an overproduction of cholesterol by the liver. Managing your heart disease will include keeping your cholesterol numbers in the normal range. You need to understand which of your cholesterol numbers are elevated, what the cause of the elevation is, and what you need to do to control it.

Cholesterol is a soft, waxy substance that is needed by the body for forming cells, making hormones, and producing bile acids needed for the digestion of fats. Most of the cholesterol needed by the body is produced by the liver.

Cholesterol is also present in the food we eat. All animal products contain cholesterol—meat, fish, poultry, dairy foods, and eggs. The average American diet includes about 600 mg of cholesterol daily. The recommended daily intake of cholesterol is less than 300 mg. Excess cholesterol circulating in the blood results in the formation of fatty plaque that can narrow arteries and cause heart attacks and strokes.

Triglycerides are another type of blood fat that is not completely understood. Increased levels of triglycerides increase the risk of coronary heart disease. A high-fat, high-cholesterol diet can raise triglyceride levels, but so can high sugar and alcohol intake.

High cholesterol and triglyceride levels in the blood result in an increased risk of coronary heart disease. The extent depends on the degree of abnormality. The Framingham Heart Study noted that individuals with a total cholesterol of 300mg/dl were twice as likely to develop coronary problems as those with cholesterol levels of 150 mg/dl. A 10 percent reduction in total cholesterol for individuals with high or moderately high cholesterol levels (greater than 200 mg/dl) decreases the risk of heart disease by 20 percent.

## Cholesterol Profile

Cholesterol and triglycerides are transported by lipoproteins to your cells. Lipoprotein surrounds the body fats with a protein coat so that it can be transported. The lipoproteins consist of LDL, HDL, and VLDL. The percent of cholesterol and/or triglycerides compared to the percent of protein defines the differences in the various lipoproteins.

*Low-density lipoprotein (LDL)* is often called "bad cholesterol" because it easily gets stuck along blood vessel walls. LDL has the greatest concentration of cholesterol. This can result in atherosclerosis, or blocked arteries.

*High-density lipoprotein (HDL)* is often called "good cholesterol" because it gathers low-density lipoproteins and transports them back to the liver to be removed from the body. HDL has the lowest concentration of cholesterol.

*Very low density lipoprotein (VLDL)* carries primarily triglycerides to other parts of the body. When it unloads the triglycerides it becomes low-density lipoprotein.

When your doctor measures your cholesterol it is called a cholesterol or lipid profile. This profile includes an analysis of the total cholesterol (a measure of free cholesterol circulating in the blood), triglycerides, HDL, LDL, and VLDL. A complete cholesterol profile is determined from blood drawn after a twelve-hour fast. A twenty-four-hour abstinence from alcohol is also recommended to provide an accurate triglyceride level. Normal values based on the National Cholesterol Education Program Guidelines are listed in Table 2.1.

**TABLE 2.1    National Cholesterol Education Program Normal Cholesterol Levels**

| CHOLESTEROL PROFILE | RECOMMENDATIONS FOR INDIVIDUALS WITH HEART DISEASE | RECOMMENDATIONS FOR INDIVIDUALS WITHOUT HEART DISEASE |
|---|---|---|
| Cholesterol | <200 | <200 |
| LDL cholesterol | <100 | <130 |
| HDL cholesterol | >35 | >35 |
| Triglycerides | <200 | <200 |
| VLDL cholesterol | <40 | <40 |

## Treatment for High Cholesterol

Treatment for elevated cholesterol will consist of three components: diet, exercise, and medication. Treatment will depend on the degree of abnormality of your cholesterol readings. The first steps will be to recommend dietary changes and introduce an exercise program. You will usually be reevaluated in three to six months. If a significant change in cholesterol numbers does not occur during this time, then medication may also be introduced. Your doctor may opt to begin medication immediately if the cholesterol numbers are extremely elevated.

## Diet

Dietary recommendations will consist of a Step I or Step II diet (see Table 2.2). If a trial period following the Step I diet is unsuccessful at lowering your cholesterol, then the more aggressive Step II diet is recommended.

**TABLE 2.2    Step I and Step II Diet Recommendations**

| DIET COMPONENT | STEP I DIET | STEP II DIET |
| --- | --- | --- |
| Cholesterol | < 300mg per day | < 200 mg per day |
| Total Fat | < 30 percent of total calories | < 25 to 30 percent of total calories |
| Saturated Fat | < 10 percent of total calories | < 7 percent of total calories |

Complete guidelines for following a low-fat, low-cholesterol diet are provided in chapter 5.

## Exercise

Regular aerobic exercise raises HDL, or "good cholesterol" levels. It lowers blood pressure, which protects the blood vessel walls. This prevents LDL cholesterol, or "bad cholesterol" from collecting along injured vessel walls. Exercise also prevents clots from forming by lowering levels of fibrinogen, which is the major clot-forming protein (see chapter 5).

## Medication

Your doctor will determine if you need medication based on the degree of the elevations of cholesterol levels, your family history, the presence of other risk factors for heart disease, and changes in your cholesterol profile after you have started a diet and exercise program.

Cholesterol medication may be prescribed based on which numbers in your cholesterol profile are abnormal (total cholesterol, HDL, LDL, or triglycerides). Cholesterol medication can act in the intestine to prevent cholesterol in food from being absorbed; it can act to prevent the formation of cholesterol in the liver; or it can interfere with the processing of cholesterol. It is important to keep in mind that cholesterol medication does not take the place of proper diet and exercise. Diet and exercise help to enhance the effectiveness of the medication. Patients often ask if it is acceptable to take an extra dose of their cholesterol medication just prior to a steak dinner; it is not. Cholesterol medication is not a diet loophole.

**REDUCING RISK:**

**CHOLESTEROL**

1.  Know your complete cholesterol profile:
    Total Cholesterol = _____
    HDL = _____
    LDL = _____
    Triglycerides = _____
    VLDL = _____

2.  Discuss with your doctor how to regain control
    of cholesterol:
    Diet
    Exercise
    Medication

3.  Educate yourself and your family about a low-fat,
    low-cholesterol diet (see chapter 5).

4.  Read food labels (see chapter 5).

5.  Exercise on a regular basis (see chapter 4).

## CALCULATING THE RISK OF HIGH BLOOD PRESSURE AND HEART DISEASE

Blood pressure is a measure of how hard your heart has to work to circulate blood through your body. The two factors that affect blood pressure are the amount of blood being pumped out of the heart (cardiac output) and the amount of resistance as the heart attempts to pump blood into the general circulation. To help you understand this better, picture water running through a narrow hose versus through a wider hose. It takes less pressure to pump water into a hose with a large diameter than it does to pump water into a hose with a small one.

At rest the heart typically beats about sixty to ninety times per minute. With each beat blood is pumped into the arteries. Arteries are the pipeline that carries blood throughout the body. They have the ability to expand and contract. An increase in resistance or volume requires a greater effort by the heart to push the blood forward into the arteries. This increased work over time causes the heart to become enlarged and less efficient. The arteries can become damaged due to scarring and loss of elasticity. This makes it more likely that cholesterol deposits will accumulate.

If you have untreated high blood pressure, you are three times more likely to have heart disease. High blood pressure also increases the risk of stroke, congestive heart failure, and kidney disease.

The brain should control blood pressure based on the body's needs. Typically, your blood pressure, heart rate, and respiratory rate will speed up or slow down to keep up with physical activity or emotional demands. If you have high blood pressure, your blood pressure may remain elevated regardless of the body's needs. The most common cause of high blood pressure, primary hypertension (the medical word for high blood pressure), is not known. Secondary hypertension is elevation of blood pressure due to the presence of another problem such as kidney disease, and is very uncommon.

## Normal Blood Pressure Readings

Most people do not understand that there is no one specific normal number for blood pressure, such as the frequently quoted 120/80. Rather, there is a range of normal blood pressure readings that includes less than 140 for systolic blood pressure (the top number) and less than 90 for diastolic blood pressure (the bottom number). The systolic reading is the highest pressure in the arteries at the time the heart contracts and pushes blood forward into the arteries.

The diastolic reading is the lowest pressure in the arteries, and represents the heart at rest between contractions. During this time the heart fills with blood and prepares for the next contraction.

## Symptoms

High blood pressure is known as the silent killer. This is because there are generally no symptoms of elevated blood pressure. The only way to know if you have elevated blood pressure is to have it measured. It is a misconception that people with high blood pressure will have headaches, nose bleeds, or flushed skin. Most people who have high blood pressure do not have any of these symptoms.

## Treatment

To treat your high blood pressure, your doctor may adjust your diet, suggest an exercise program, and/or prescribe medication.

## Diet

If you are overweight, you are three times more likely to have high blood pressure than those who are not overweight. Therefore, following recommended guidelines in the weight management section of this chapter will help with blood pressure control.

The amount of sodium you should consume in your diet to maintain health and a normal hydration state continues to be studied. Your doctor may recommend that you restrict your sodium intake because research indicates that some individuals may be sensitive to sodium. Excess sodium causes fluid retention, and may increase artery constriction, resulting in high blood pressure. For individuals with high blood pressure, the American Heart Association recommends restricting daily sodium intake to less than 2,400 mg daily. This involves avoiding adding salt to foods, eating fresh fruits and vegetables, and monitoring milligrams of sodium noted on food labels, particularly in processed foods.

# BLOOD PRESSURE CLASSIFICATIONS AND RECOMMENDATIONS

**SYSTOLIC:**

- <130 mm Hg: normal blood pressure; recheck within 2 years
- 130–139 mm Hg: high normal; recheck within 1 year
- 140–159 mm Hg: mild hypertension; confirm within 2 months
- 160–179 mm Hg: moderate hypertension; see doctor within 1 month
- 180–209 mm Hg: severe hypertension; see doctor within 1 week
- 210 mm Hg or higher: very severe hypertension; see doctor immediately

**DIASTOLIC:**

- <85 mm Hg: normal blood pressure; recheck within 2 years
- 85–89 mm Hg: high normal blood pressure; recheck within 1 year
- 90–99 mm Hg: mild hypertension; confirm within 2 months
- 100–109 mm Hg: moderate hypertension; see doctor within 1 month
- 110–119 mm Hg: severe hypertension; see doctor within 1 week
- 120 mm Hg or higher: very severe hypertension; see doctor immediately

*Source: 1993 Report of the Joint National Committee on Detection, Evaluation, and Treatment of High Blood Pressure.*

Excessive caffeine consumption can also cause an increase in blood pressure. The recommended daily maximum amount of caffeine is 200 mg per day, or the equivalent of two 8-ounce cups of coffee daily. (See Table 2.3 below.)

**TABLE 2.3    How Much Caffeine Do You Consume?**

| FOOD OR DRINK | SERVING SIZE | CAFFEINE (MG) |
|---|---|---|
| Brewed coffee | 6 oz. | 83 |
| Instant coffee | 6 oz. | 60 |
| Decaffeinated coffee | 6 oz. | 3 |
| Leaf tea | 6 oz. | 41 |
| Instant tea | 6 oz. | 28 |
| Colas | 12 oz. | 40–72 |
| Cocoa | 6 oz. | 10 |
| Chocolate | 1 oz. | 5–10 |
| Excedrin | 1 tablet | 66 |
| Anacin | 1 tablet | 32 |

## Exercise

Exercise allows the body to function at a lower blood pressure, which can reduce stress on the arteries. Exercise can also strengthen the heart muscle so it can pump more blood with each beat. A regular aerobic exercise program will provide you with both short- and long-term benefits. The short-term benefit of exercise is lower blood pressure after exercise that is sustained for several hours. The long-term benefit of aerobic exercise performed three to five times per week has been reported to include a 7-point drop in systolic blood pressure and a 6-point drop in diastolic blood pressure.

Exercise also helps with weight and stress management, which directly helps to control blood pressure. A recommended exercise program is described in detail in chapter 4.

## Medication

If your blood pressure cannot be consistently controlled with diet and exercise, your doctor may choose to prescribe medication. Treatment with medication depends on your specific medical history, but will be generally considered when systolic blood pressure readings are consistently greater than 160 and diastolic readings are consistently greater than 100. Common medication options include:

1. *Diuretics:* flush excess water and salt out of your system to maintain a normal fluid volume status.
2. *Beta blockers:* alter the way hormones control blood pressure and reduce the force of the heartbeat.
3. *Vasodilators:* relax the blood vessels.
4. *Calcium channel blockers:* interfere with the flow of calcium in and out of cells, resulting in relaxation of blood vessels and lower blood pressures.
5. *ACE inhibitors:* prevent chemical reactions, resulting in lower blood pressure.

## CALCULATING THE RISK OF SMOKING AND HEART DISEASE

Stopping smoking is the single most important step you can take to improve your health and decrease the risk of complications from heart disease.

If you smoke, you are twice as likely to develop heart disease as a nonsmoker. The more you smoke, the higher your risk of heart disease, and smoking is the leading cause of preventable death. No one

**REDUCING RISK:**
**HIGH BLOOD PRESSURE**

1. Record your blood pressure at various times of the day.
2. Discuss abnormal readings with your doctor.
3. Maintain your ideal body weight.
4. Exercise aerobically three to five times per week (with your doctors' approval).
5. Limit sodium intake to 2,400 mg daily.
6. Limit caffeine intake to two 8-ounce servings daily.
7. Take prescribed medication as directed by your doctor.

disputes that smoking jeopardizes your health. However, smoking is a challenging behavior to change because the nicotine in cigarettes is physically addicting and smoking is a habit-forming behavior.

Smoking has both temporary and long-term effects on your body. There are 4,000 potentially harmful substances in tobacco. The immediate impact of just one cigarette includes an increase in heart rate, blood pressure, and demand for oxygen. It causes your blood vessels to constrict and carbon monoxide, a by-product of cigarettes, gets into the blood and reduces the amount of oxygen your blood can carry to body tissues. This greater demand for oxygen and decreased supply can increase the incidence of angina.

The long-term effects of smoking include a lowering of the HDL or good cholesterol and damage to the lining of blood vessel walls which increase the risk of plaque formation. In addition to increasing your risk for heart disease, smoking increases your chance of lung disease, a variety of cancers, stroke, and peripheral vascular disease.

## What to Expect After You Quit

Smokers struggle with the physical and psychological behaviors related to smoking. However, you *can* quit smoking. The benefits of quitting will be noticed immediately. These include:

### Health Benefits

- Lower heart rate, blood pressure.
- Relaxation of blood vessels.
- Decreased frequency of angina.
- Elimination of smoker's cough.
- Decreased risk of cancer including lung, esophagus, mouth, throat, pancreas, kidney, bladder, and cervix.
- Decreased risk of lung disease including bronchitis and emphysema.
- Decreased risk of heart disease.
- Improved life span.

### Lifestyle Benefits

- Improved body odor and breath odor.
- Improved sense of smell and taste.
- Reduced teeth and fingernail stains.
- Fewer skin wrinkles.
- Improved financial status.

Quitting smoking will not be easy. Nicotine is an addictive substance, and symptoms appear upon its withdrawal. You may experience irritability, restlessness, anxiety, insomnia, and impatience. Additionally, smoking is a habit-forming behavior that requires planned strategies to change.

## STRATEGIES TO QUIT SMOKING

There are a variety of approaches to kicking the habit of smoking. You will need to evaluate what works best for you based on your previous experience with change. Do you prefer to do this with a group or would you rather go it alone? The following is a list of some strategies to quit smoking:

- *Quitting "cold turkey."* This is a strategy that many have used successfully. Select a quit date, remove all smoking materials from the environment, and rally the support of your family and friends by telling them you are quitting. If you have tried to quit in the past, use this experience to identify what worked and what didn't. It will also help to take note of times when you are most likely to smoke and develop strategies to prevent smoking at these times. Many organizations such as the American Cancer Society, the American Lung Association, and the American Heart Association have materials that will help you to quit smoking. These groups are listed in appendix A.
- *Medication.* Medication is prescribed with caution for individuals with known heart disease. Nicotine replacement therapy (patches or gum) has many of the same effects on the cardiovascular system as smoking itself. Consult with your doctor to determine if these are good options for you. There are many smoking cessation remedies that do not require a doctor's prescription; however, do not use any of these without first consulting with your health care provider.
- *Behavior modification.* Offered through support groups or individual counseling, behavior modification can help you identify why you smoke and find substitutes for situations in which you normally do so. Additionally, in group programs, the peer support offered to members can be helpful.
- *Hypnosis.* For some individuals, hypnosis has been successful. Sessions may be private or part of a group smoking cessation program.

## A NOTE ABOUT WEIGHT GAIN

Many smokers hesitate to quit because of concern about gaining weight. You may gain a small amount of weight for a variety of reasons. Weight gain may be caused by using food as a substitute for cigarettes. Using gum, carrot and celery sticks, and hard candy may help to prevent weight gain. Nicotine causes a slight increase in metabolism; thus, when you stop taking in nicotine, your metabolism slows. The same amount of food could cause a small weight gain. In addition, as you quit smoking, you will probably experience improved taste and smell, and with this an improved appetite. But most research demonstrates that the average weight gain is about 5 pounds, which is negligible compared to the health risks of smoking.

## Secondhand Smoke

Individuals exposed to cigarette smoke take in many of the same toxins that are being inhaled by the smoker. These toxins include carbon monoxide, tar, and nicotine. They have many of the same effects on these individuals as they do on the smoker. Secondhand smoke has been linked to the development of heart and lung disease and causes complications for individuals already experiencing these problems.

## CALCULATING THE RISK OF DIABETES AND HEART DISEASE

Diabetes mellitus is a disease that results in increased levels of sugar in the blood. In the healthy individual, the pancreas produces insulin, which transports sugar to the cells to be used for energy. With diabetes, the pancreas stops producing insulin, or the body becomes resistant to using insulin properly.

**REDUCING RISK:**

**SMOKING**

1.  Set a quit date.
2.  Rally support of family and friends by letting them know your intentions to quit.
3.  Clear your environment of cigarettes and other smoking supplies.
4.  Review past quit attempts and evaluate what worked and what didn't.
5.  Discuss with your doctor the need for nicotine patches during early withdrawal.
6.  Consider a support group or individual counseling to bolster your efforts.

Type I diabetes is caused by diminished or absent production of insulin by the pancreas. This is often referred to as "juvenile onset diabetes" because it is commonly seen in younger people, although individuals can be diagnosed with Type I diabetes at any age. Type II diabetes is caused by the body developing a resistance to insulin. The insulin no longer properly transports sugar to the cells, resulting in high blood sugar levels. Type II diabetes is commonly seen in overweight middle-aged adults and individuals with a family history of diabetes. It is the most common cause of diabetes and affects as many as 7 million adults. Many more are unaware that they have this disease.

Uncontrolled diabetes promotes the development of heart disease. The increase in circulating blood sugar present in diabetes results in damage to blood vessels, increasing the likelihood that plaque will collect along vessel lining walls and will lead to narrowing of the coronary arteries. In addition to doubling your risk of heart disease, diabetes increases your risk of stroke and peripheral vascular disease (narrowing of the vessels of your legs due to plaque formation). Diabetes can also cause damage to the kidneys, eyes, and nervous system.

## Special Consideration: Diabetes and Heart Disease

If you have diabetes and heart disease, be aware that your heart disease symptoms may differ from the general population. You may not feel chest pain or angina, or the symptoms may be very mild due to damage or loss of sensitivity of nerve endings from the diabetes. Therefore, if you experience any symptoms such as fatigue, shortness of breath, or minor or intermittent chest, arm, jaw, or back pain, this may signal a more serious problem. They should be brought to your doctor's immediate attention. It is also very important that you receive regular follow-up testing to identify problems for which you may have no symptoms at all.

Preventing the progression of heart disease will be achieved by maintaining normal blood sugar levels. You should own a blood sugar monitor and check blood sugar levels as directed by your doctor. This may include checking levels as frequently as four times daily until they are consistently showing a normal trend. Achieving the right dose and timing of medication may require some adjustments as you make changes in diet and exercise routines.

Exercise helps the body use insulin more efficiently. Guidance from a health professional when starting an exercise program will help you tailor your exercise program, diet, and medication based on your response to activity. When beginning a program, it may be necessary to check blood sugar levels before and after exercise to determine its effect.

Aggressive management of your other cardiac risk factors will be particularly important to help balance the effects of diabetes. This should include maintaining your ideal weight, cholesterol, and blood pressure levels, quitting smoking if you currently do so, and taking part in a regular exercise program.

**REDUCING RISK:**

**DIABETES**

1. Purchase a home glucose monitor and monitor daily blood sugar levels as directed by your doctor. Inform your doctor of elevated readings and treat as directed.
2. Maintain your ideal body weight.
3. Follow dietary guidelines as prescribed by your doctor. Consider evaluation with a registered dietitian.
4. Maintain normal cholesterol levels.
5. Maintain normal blood pressure.
6. Exercise three to five times per week following guidelines for individuals with diabetes (see chapter 4).
7. Stop smoking.

## CALCULATING THE RISK OF PHYSICAL INACTIVITY AND HEART DISEASE

Regular physical activity decreases your chances of heart disease and helps to control other cardiac risk factors including blood pressure, HDL cholesterol, diabetes, obesity, and stress. If you have heart disease, aerobic exercise can decrease the incidence of complications; and if you do have a second heart attack, your history of regular exercise improves survival and limits complications.

Aerobic exercise is recommended to improve cardiovascular health. It increases heart rate and breathing rate, tones and strengthens muscles, and improves how the body uses oxygen for energy. It trains your heart to do its work more efficiently. Examples of aerobic exercise are walking, jogging, bicycling, swimming, and rowing.

Try to look at exercise as an opportunity, not drudgery. It is your opportunity to do something good for yourself. Exercising on a regular basis will help to improve your fitness level and overall health. Being physically active throughout the day in addition to your aerobic exercise program will also help to maintain your fitness level. This can include walking the stairs rather than taking the elevator, parking at the far end of a grocery store lot, gardening, walking the dog, and so on. Chapter 4 provides the basis for developing and maintaining an exercise program, after your doctor has given you approval to begin doing so.

If you have heart disease, you should receive clearance from your doctor to begin exercising. Usually a stress test is performed to determine the exact level of activity that is safe for you. This test monitors your heart rate and rhythm while you walk on a treadmill. The intensity is gradually increased until you reach a maximum heart rate level. This helps the doctor determine what exercise level is safe for you based on how your heart rate, heart rhythm, and blood pressure respond.

Your doctor may recommend a medically supervised cardiac rehabilitation program during the early stages of your recovery. Hospitals throughout the country offer these programs, which introduce exercise based on your specific medical history. During your exercise session your heart rate, heart rhythm, and blood pressure response to exercise is monitored by specially trained health professionals. These programs also include an education program on living with heart disease.

**REDUCING RISK:**
**EXERCISE**

1. Discuss your exercise program with your doctor.
2. Plan to exercise on a regular basis (see chapter 4).
3. Listen to your body and stop exercise if you begin to feel ill. Notify your doctor of any unusual symptoms occurring during exercise.
4. Do not exercise if you are sick or injured.
5. Ask your doctor about how often you need to repeat your stress test.

## CALCULATING THE RISK:
## OBESITY AND HEART DISEASE

Almost all of us at one time or another have put on a few more pounds than we would like. At what point does excess weight adversely affect our health? Scientists continue to study this subject. However, research consistently shows that being overweight increases your risk for developing heart disease and for complications when heart disease is already present. It is not certain if obesity independently increases the risk for heart disease, or if the adverse health effects of obesity that include diabetes, hypertension, and high cholesterol are the reason heart disease develops when you are overweight.

The impact of obesity on overall health is substantial. In addition to heart disease, being overweight (greater than 20 percent above recommended weight) makes you twice as likely to have elevated cholesterol and triglyceride levels, three times more likely to have diabetes, and three times more likely to have elevated blood pressure. You are also more likely to have back and joint problems and gallbladder disease, and you are at increased risk for stroke.

There are a variety of ways to determine if you are overweight. The most commonly used methods are height and weight tables, Body Mass Index, and location of fat distribution. Height and weight tables provide a general guide for appropriate weight based on gender and body type. Tables 2.4 and 2.5 present weights based on research that identifies weight ranges that promote favorable life expectancies.

**TABLE 2.4**     **Ideal Height and Weight Ranges**

| HEIGHT | WEIGHT IN POUNDS |
|--------|------------------|
| 4'10"  | 91–119           |
| 4'11"  | 94–124           |
| 5'0"   | 97–128           |
| 5'1"   | 101–132          |
| 5'2"   | 104–137          |
| 5'3"   | 107–141          |
| 5'4"   | 111–146          |
| 5'5"   | 114–150          |
| 5'6"   | 118–155          |
| 5'7"   | 121–160          |
| 5'8"   | 125–164          |
| 5'9"   | 129–169          |
| 5'10"  | 132–174          |
| 5'11"  | 136–179          |
| 6'0"   | 140–184          |

*Source: U.S. Department of Agriculture and the Department of Health and Human Services. Weight Guidelines for Adults, 1995.*

TABLE 2.5   Body Weight in Pounds According to Height and Body Mass Index

BODY MASS INDEX

| Height (inches) | Body Weight (Pounds) 19 | 20 | 21 | 22 | 23 | 24 | 25 | 26 | 27 | 28 | 29 | 30 | 35 | 40 |
|---|---|---|---|---|---|---|---|---|---|---|---|---|---|---|
| 58 | 91 | 96 | 100 | 105 | 110 | 115 | 119 | 124 | 129 | 134 | 138 | 143 | 167 | 191 |
| 59 | 94 | 96 | 104 | 109 | 114 | 119 | 124 | 128 | 133 | 138 | 143 | 148 | 173 | 198 |
| 60 | 97 | 99 | 107 | 112 | 118 | 123 | 128 | 133 | 138 | 143 | 148 | 153 | 179 | 204 |
| 61 | 100 | 102 | 111 | 116 | 122 | 127 | 132 | 139 | 143 | 148 | 153 | 158 | 185 | 211 |
| 62 | 104 | 106 | 115 | 120 | 126 | 131 | 136 | 142 | 147 | 153 | 158 | 164 | 191 | 218 |
| 63 | 107 | 109 | 118 | 124 | 130 | 135 | 141 | 146 | 152 | 158 | 163 | 169 | 197 | 225 |
| 64 | 110 | 113 | 122 | 128 | 134 | 140 | 145 | 151 | 159 | 163 | 169 | 174 | 204 | 232 |

| | | | | | | | | | | | | | | |
|---|---|---|---|---|---|---|---|---|---|---|---|---|---|---|
| 65 | 114 | 116 | 126 | 132 | 138 | 144 | 150 | 158 | 162 | 168 | 174 | 180 | 210 | 240 |
| 66 | 118 | 120 | 130 | 136 | 142 | 148 | 155 | 161 | 167 | 173 | 179 | 186 | 216 | 247 |
| 67 | 121 | 124 | 134 | 140 | 146 | 153 | 159 | 166 | 172 | 178 | 185 | 191 | 223 | 255 |
| 68 | 125 | 127 | 138 | 144 | 151 | 158 | 164 | 171 | 177 | 184 | 190 | 197 | 230 | 262 |
| 69 | 128 | 131 | 142 | 149 | 155 | 162 | 169 | 176 | 182 | 189 | 196 | 203 | 236 | 270 |
| 70 | 132 | 135 | 146 | 153 | 160 | 167 | 174 | 181 | 188 | 195 | 202 | 207 | 243 | 278 |
| 71 | 136 | 139 | 150 | 157 | 165 | 172 | 179 | 186 | 193 | 200 | 208 | 215 | 250 | 286 |
| 72 | 140 | 143 | 154 | 162 | 169 | 177 | 184 | 191 | 199 | 206 | 213 | 221 | 258 | 294 |
| 73 | 144 | 147 | 159 | 166 | 174 | 182 | 189 | 197 | 204 | 212 | 219 | 227 | 265 | 302 |
| 74 | 148 | 151 | 163 | 171 | 179 | 186 | 194 | 202 | 210 | 218 | 225 | 233 | 272 | 311 |
| 75 | 152 | 155 | 168 | 176 | 184 | 192 | 200 | 208 | 216 | 224 | 232 | 240 | 279 | 319 |
| 76 | 156 | 160 | 172 | 180 | 189 | 197 | 205 | 213 | 221 | 230 | 238 | 246 | 287 | 328 |

Body Mass Index (BMI = Weight (kg) / Height (m)²) is useful in identifying whether your weight places you at increased risk for heart disease. To figure out your Body Mass Index, use the following formula (or see Table 2.5):

$$\text{BMI} = \frac{\text{weight in kilograms (total pounds} \div 2.2)}{\text{height in meters 2 } (\sqrt{\text{total inches}} \times 2.5 \div 100)}$$

Research indicates that individuals with a body mass index greater than 27 have an increased risk of heart disease. The ideal body mass index of 22 to 25 is associated with the lowest mortality.

Fat distribution is another measure of obesity as it relates to the development of heart disease. In lower-body obesity (pear shape), your fat is distributed in the hips and thighs. Central obesity (apple shape) refers to fat distributions in the abdomen and trunk. If you have an apple shape, you have a higher risk for developing heart disease. Fat stored in the abdomen is more active than fat in other parts of the body. The fatty breakdown gets into the circulation and may result in increased levels of cholesterol. To determine your shape, measure your waist and hip girth at the widest point. If your waist girth is greater than hip girth, you are an apple shape. A ratio of less than .8 is desirable for women, and less than 1.0 is desirable for men.

## How Can I Lose Weight?

Your weight loss plan should focus on the simple formula of decreasing calorie intake and increasing calories burned through a more active lifestyle and regular aerobic exercise. Anyone who has attempted a weight loss program knows that it is more complicated than this. Dealing with the emotional aspects of why you eat, finding the time to exercise, and developing an interest in shopping and preparing healthy foods can be a challenge to all of us. A sensible approach to weight loss will focus on achieving a weight loss of 1 to 2 pounds per week. This will require reduced calorie intake, a low-fat diet, and exercise. You will succeed by following these steps:

### Step 1: Determine Dietary Calorie Needs
Begin by determining daily calorie needs.

Desirable weight = _____

Desirable weight x (Activity Factor)* = _____ Calories per day
> *Factor 13: Sedentary lifestyle = almost no exercise
> *Factor 15: Active lifestyle = moderate exercise 20 minutes three to five times per week
> *Factor 17: Very active = 1 hour exercise five to six times per week

Calories per day – 500 = Calories per day to achieve 1-pound weight loss per week

*Example:*
> Jane is a forty-five-year-old woman who is 5'4" and weighs 186 pounds. Her ideal weight is 146 pounds (body mass index of 25). Her short-term weight loss goal is 12 pounds over the next three months, which is a 1-pound weight loss per week. She currently exercises aerobically three times per week at a health club for forty-five minutes.

> Desirable weight = 146 pounds
> Desirable weight x Activity Factor 15 = 2,190 calories per day
> 2,190 (calories per day) – 500 (reduction in calories to lose 1 pound per week) = 1,690
> 1,690 calories per day to lose 1 pound per week

### Step 2: Modify Dietary Fat Intake
Fat intake in your diet should not exceed 30 percent of your total calories, and some experts recommend that in the presence of heart disease, no more than 20 percent of your total calories should come from fat. Each fat gram is equal to 9 calories (compared to 4 calories

for carbohydrates and protein). The following table recommends maximum fat grams based on total calories consumed to maintain a diet with less than 20 or 30 percent total calories from fat. (See Table 2.6.)

TABLE 2.6    Daily Fat Intake by Calorie Level

| TOTAL CALORIE LEVEL (calories/day) | 20% TOTAL CALORIES FROM FAT PER DAY (grams/day) | 30% TOTAL CALORIES FROM FAT PER DAY (grams/day) | MAXIMUM SATURATED FAT (grams/day) |
|---|---|---|---|
| 1,000 | 22 | 33 | 11 |
| 1,200 | 26 | 40 | 13 |
| 1,400 | 31 | 47 | 15 |
| 1,600 | 36 | 53 | 17 |
| 1,800 | 40 | 60 | 20 |
| 2,000 | 44 | 67 | 22 |
| 2,200 | 49 | 73 | 24 |
| 2,400 | 53 | 80 | 26 |
| 2,600 | 58 | 87 | 28 |
| 2,800 | 62 | 93 | 30 |
| 3,000 | 67 | 100 | 32 |

You will achieve an overall well-balanced diet by eating three meals daily that include a variety of foods in reasonable portion sizes. This diet should include protein, dairy products, and especially vegetables, fruits, and grains. Chapter 5 describes in detail strategies for making dietary changes and selecting a weight loss program that will work for you.

### Step 3: Exercise Regularly

Exercise requires your body to work harder, which uses more calories. After you stop exercising, your body continues to burn calories at an increased rate for a few hours. The long-term effect of exercise is that your proportion of body fat decreases while the proportion of lean muscle mass increases. The more lean muscle you have, the higher your calorie expenditure will be. Muscle burns more calories than fat.

Exercise guidelines to promote weight loss involve a slightly different strategy than for general health maintenance. While trying to lose weight, you should gradually increase your exercise frequency to five times per week. Your exercise should be completed at a lower intensity range (60 percent of the target heart rate range). Exercise should be sustained at this level for thirty to sixty minutes. During the first twenty minutes of exercise your body is using stored carbohydrates and circulating fat for energy. After approximately twenty minutes, the body begins to burn stored fat for energy. Complete details on developing a safe exercise program are presented in chapter 4.

## A Note About Medication

The most successful weight loss program is one that makes long-term adjustments in calorie intake and expenditure through moderate dietary changes and exercise. Use of medication to aid weight loss has recently gained attention. These medications usually suppress carbohydrate cravings by affecting appetite and mood. These and all weight loss products continue to be controversial due to side effects and questionable long-term effectiveness. Careful discussion with your doctor should precede any use of weight loss products.

**REDUCING RISK:**
**OBESITY**

1. Review Body Mass Index/Height and Weight tables.
2. Set a goal weight.
3. Determine your daily required calorie fat gram intake.
4. Gradually increase aerobic exercise to five times per week for thirty to sixty minutes at 60 percent of the target heart rate range (see chapter 4).
5. Review previous weight loss attempts and anticipate challenges.
6. Evaluate your need for a structured program and/or support group.

## CALCULATING THE RISK OF STRESS AND HEART DISEASE

Stress by definition is our emotional, behavioral, physical, and mental response to life's experiences. Stress is good (eustress) when it heightens our mental acuity to meet the challenge of experiences such as giving a speech, taking an examination, or interviewing for a job.

Stress becomes harmful (distress) when day-to-day activities trigger a stress response. Over time, the stress response evolved as a heightened awareness to danger, eliciting a "fight or flight" reaction. Stress to our ancestors was coming face to face with a mountain lion while on a hunting expedition. The physiologic change necessary to meet this danger was a release of hormones that caused an increase in heart rate, blood pressure, muscle tension, blood clotting, blood vessel constriction, and increased blood flow to the brain and muscles. However, this life-threatening occurrence happened only rarely in a lifetime.

Now review what you see as stress in the twentieth century: traffic jams, football games, credit card bills, a missed appointment, or a disagreement with your spouse. Stress is a risk factor for you if routine events such as daily work and family responsibilities and social activities elicit the stress response several times during the course of a day. If we allow the stress response to occur, we suddenly have an increase in heart rate, blood pressure, breathing rate, and muscle tension most of the time. Eventually this causes wear and tear on our cardiovascular system.

The physiologic response to stress can cause an increase in frequency of angina episodes, elevated blood pressure, and an increased risk of plaque formation due to damage to blood vessel walls. It is estimated that this risk factor alone can double your chances of heart disease.

## Determining Your Stress Triggers

Studies by cardiologists Meyer Friedman and Ray Rosenman in the 1970s defined personality types as Type A and Type B. Individuals displaying predominantly Type A personality traits were found to be at increased risk for developing heart disease. These traits include time urgency, eating fast, speaking rapidly, impatience, competitiveness, easily upset or angered, highly motivated to achieve, and often perceived as strong and forceful. Type B behavior was less likely to contribute to heart disease. These individuals display personality traits that include moving unhurriedly, eating slowly, speaking slowly, and being patient, cooperative, and collaborative.

More recently it has been suggested that the more serious problem may be if these Type A traits are a result of cynicism, anger, and hostility to the outside environment. One study, the Multiple Risk Factor Intervention Trial, noted that hostility doubles the risk of heart attack in middle-aged men.

With your goal of preventing further progression of heart disease, you need to take an inventory of situations, perceptions, and behaviors that inappropriately trigger the stress response in you. Chapter 6 will outline how to practice successful stress management. You will complete a stress symptom checklist, learn to recognize the warning signs of stress, and identify and develop strategies to assist you in keeping control of your stress response. You do not need to totally eliminate stress in your life. Rather, you want to be in control of stress rather than letting it control you.

**REDUCING RISK:**
**STRESS**

1. Complete the stress symptom checklist in chapter 6.
2. Identify perceptions and personality traits that increase stress in your life.
3. Recognize the warning signs of stress.
4. Develop strategies to improve emotional, behavioral, and physical response to stressful situations (see chapter 6).
5. Obtain professional counseling if independent efforts at stress management are not successful.

## UNCONTROLLABLE
## CARDIAC RISK FACTORS

Age, family history, and gender are three risk factors that you cannot change. The healthy lifestyle choices you make will help to balance these risk factors. Since coronary artery disease is progressive, involving the buildup of plaque, it makes sense that as you get older you're at greater risk for heart disease. The degenerative effects of aging, including aging of the vessel lining walls, also make it more likely that plaque will collect. In addition, the long-term effects of other risk factors including high blood pressure, obesity, smoking, stress, elevated cholesterol, and an inactive lifestyle catch up with us in our older years (if not sooner!).

If you have a parent, grandparent, or sibling who developed heart disease before age fifty-five in men and before age sixty-five in women, then you may have a genetic predisposition to heart disease. High cholesterol, high blood pressure, diabetes, and obesity all may have a genetic link that could put us at increased risk for heart disease. Additionally, race may increase your risk. African Americans have higher incidences of diabetes and high blood pressure.

Heart disease is the leading cause of death for men and women. Gender is an issue because men are more likely to develop heart disease at younger ages than women. The female hormone estrogen may protect women before menopause. After menopause, the incidence of heart disease in women equals that of men. As mentioned previously, however, making healthy lifestyle choices will help to balance these risk factors.

### A Special Note to Women

In the 1990s, more women than men are dying of heart disease. Women mistakenly believe that breast cancer is their most serious health threat. This misunderstanding may result in ignoring symptoms that, if reported, may mean early treatment of heart disease.

Women are different. They have risk factors that are specific to women only; their symptoms signaling heart disease may be different; the female anatomy and physiology is different; diagnostic testing may require special considerations; and treatment for women all needs to be tailored to these differences.

Women have many of the same risk factors as men, including obesity, high cholesterol, stress, hypertension, inactive lifestyle, diabetes, and smoking. Additional risks that are different from men include the following:

- Use of oral contraceptives.
- Elevations in triglycerides are a stronger risk than for men.
- Menopause causes a decrease in estrogen and an increase in heart disease in women.

Symptoms of heart disease may present differently in women than in men. Symptoms may be more subtle, such as mild chest pain or tightness, or throat or jaw pain. Shortness of breath, chronic fatigue, ankle swelling, and/or nausea or indigestion should be discussed with your doctor.

Female anatomical differences include a higher percentage of body fat, a smaller heart, and smaller coronary arteries. These make traditional diagnostic procedures less reliable. Many research studies to determine effective means to diagnose and treat heart disease were completed on men and may not be as accurate for women. Stress testing has been determined to be less reliable for women than for men. A more accurate test may be the thallium stress test, which uses cardiac perfusion imaging to visualize the heart. Echocardiograms, which transmit sound waves that produce an image of the heart, may not always be able to transmit through breast tissue. The message to women is that if undiagnosed symptoms persist, they should inquire about additional testing regardless of previous normal test results.

Treatment for heart disease in women should include consideration of hormone replacement therapy. The female hormone estrogen causes an increase in HDL ("good cholesterol") that corresponds to a delay in development of heart disease in women before menopause, and may prevent progression of heart disease. Therefore, all postmenopausal women should discuss hormone replacement therapy with their doctors. Other treatment may include medication and interventions including angioplasty, stent, and coronary bypass surgery. This treatment correlates to that offered to men; however, special consideration needs to be made for women's size, heart size, and smaller coronary arteries.

## MOVING FORWARD

By now you know what work needs to be done in terms of personal lifestyle changes. Some of these changes may seem natural to you; others may be more of a challenge. Your first job is to identify and prioritize alterations that need to be made. When you can do this you are on your way to recovery. As part of this process, begin to recognize your feelings; they may include anger, fear, or resentment. Then figure out how you will channel this energy toward accomplishing more beneficial goals.

Recovering from heart disease is a journey. Experimenting will help you discover what works for you and what doesn't. Draw on every internal and external resource you have to make all of this work. What has helped you get through difficult situations in the past . . . family, friends, humor, or an invigorating workout? You may realize by now that healing is a process, not an end point. Keep moving forward!

§

## CHAPTER THREE

# ADJUSTING TO YOUR NEW LIFESTYLE

THE CHALLENGE OF YOUR RECOVERY WILL BE TO RETURN TO AN optimal state of physical, spiritual, mental, social, and emotional health. As you begin the healing process, think about the value you place on each of these dimensions. The health-conscious behaviors you subsequently choose to adopt will be influenced by these attitudes and beliefs.

## COPING WITH YOUR ILLNESS

Adjusting to your new lifestyle requires establishing priorities and goals. View this time as an opportunity to make decisions that will positively affect your health. Some people feel overwhelmed in the beginning. The aim of this chapter is to provide information that will assist you during this transition. We will discuss issues that will help you to move forward: handling the emotional impacts of illness, managing family concerns, returning to work, and understanding activity limitations and concerns related to intimacy.

## The Emotional Impacts of Illness

It all happens so fast! One day you are living life normally, and the next your usual routine is completely disrupted. Suddenly everything that was once the norm is no longer so. Your medical care team worked hard to find the right combination of treatments and medication to stabilize your condition. For your part, you were told you need to make changes in your life to reduce your risk of future health problems. From this point on you feel changed in some way. Some people have described their reactions to being diagnosed with heart disease in the following ways:

- "One minute I was laughing and playing with the kids and the next thing I knew I had had surgery and was afraid to pick up my child."
- "I've always been the one that my family depends on and now I have to depend on them."
- "I used to think I would easily live to ninety years old, but now I'm not so sure."
- "I used to be confident in doing things and now I'm afraid to try anything new."
- "Can I make all the lifestyle changes my doctor has advised?"
- "I wonder if I can return to work again."
- "I feel that resuming sexual relations will change in some way—now that I've had a heart attack."

Did you wonder if you were going to live through this crisis? You may still feel vulnerable. Now you must learn to face unknowns and uncertainties about your health, status, your family life, returning to work, and resuming sexual relations.

You may experience a sense of helplessness, inadequacy, and

dependence immediately following being diagnosed with heart disease. You may find yourself incapable of handling the day-to-day pressures of life. These are normal responses. It is common for you to want to retreat or withdraw from this situation because it feels safe to do so. As you experience improvements in your physical health, you will transition away from these emotional turmoils and toward feeling increased confidence in your future health status and quality of life. Although the unknowns and the reminders of your vulnerability (ongoing treatments and the need for medications) still exist, you will begin to feel less vulnerable and more independent as time passes and you come to terms with your illness.

When a crisis is upon you, a natural defense mechanism is to deny the seriousness of the problem. This period of denial may allow you time to gradually adapt to being diagnosed with heart disease. Denial, however, provides only temporary relief from distress. Denial is often followed by one or more of these feelings: anxiety, fear of death, loss of confidence, anger, and depression. These emotions can be brought on by the need for lifestyle changes involving diet, career, family roles, and other activities. Knowing what to expect and how to confront these emotions may help to relieve the emotional impact of illness and ease the transition to your new life.

### *Confront Your Fears*
You may be experiencing a number of different types of fear, such as fear of losing control, fear of dependency, and fear of death. Confronting each of these involves shifting your focus from feeling out of control, helpless, and vulnerable to recognizing your fears, discussing them openly with family and friends, and identifying coping strategies. These actions will lessen the intensity of these fears. Follow these guidelines as you confront your fears:

1. Avoid suppressing your fears. Talk to someone who will understand. Discuss unpleasant and painful topics openly.
2. Use exercise as a tool to release tensions.

3. Practice relaxation techniques regularly to rid yourself of everyday tensions (see chapter 6).

4. Visualize success in meeting the physical and emotional challenges of living with heart disease.

### Confront Your Anger

Anger is common when you are first diagnosed with heart disease. You may be angry at yourself, thinking that perhaps something you did caused your illness. You may be mad because you have always led a healthy lifestyle and still developed heart disease, or feel you are losing control over your lifestyle choices. Whatever the reason(s), try not to become overwhelmed. It is normal to feel angry at times, but when it occurs too often, lasts too long, begins to intensify, and disrupts your behavior, it becomes problematic and can affect your physical and emotional health. Avoid keeping anger bottled up inside, releasing it in an aggressive manner, and becoming upset over trivial concerns. These are all ineffective ways to manage your anger. Follow these guidelines as you confront your anger:

1. Identify what it is you are angry about. Develop a plan to resolve this conflict.

2. Avoid suppressing your anger. Learn to release your anger in safe and healthy ways, such as talking to someone who will understand.

3. Be prepared for tense moments. What action will you take to diffuse the situation?

4. Be aware of your physical and behavioral changes caused by anger (for example, flushed feeling in your face, increased heart rate, increased rate of speech, tense muscles, distorted thoughts). When you feel this happening, try to resolve your anger in a constructive way.

5. Avoid lashing out at family or friends who are not the primary source of your anger. Use them to obtain support and comfort, not as your victims.

As you begin to manage your anger, you will find yourself in better spirits and feeling more relaxed.

### Confront Your Depression

Depression is a common reaction to being diagnosed with a chronic illness. It may be part of your emotional response to the situation. However, it may also be a side effect of certain cardiac medications such as beta blockers, blood pressure medications, and some medications for irregular heart rhythms. (These drugs are discussed in detail in chapter 7.)

Common symptoms of depression include social withdrawal, diminished appetite, sleeplessness, lack of energy, inability to make decisions, and tearfulness. Remember, some amount of depression is normal. However, when symptoms such as these become unmanageable or continue for prolonged periods, it is important that they be discussed with your doctor immediately. Untreated depression can result in delays in recovery. To assist you in dealing with symptoms of depression, follow these suggestions:

1. Set achievable goals each day and accomplish them.
2. Continue your morning routine as you did prior to feeling depressed (for example, get out of bed, shower, and dress each day).
3. Eat three meals daily, selecting foods from all food groups. Avoid high-sugar snacks.
4. Exercise three to five times per week.
5. Practice relaxation techniques.
6. Avoid suppressing your feelings. Talk to someone who will understand.
7. Seek psychological counseling if you are struggling to overcome the symptoms of depression on your own.

Emotional responses to illness can quickly sap your energy if you let them. Try not to suppress them, or let them run wild. If they remain or intensify, they can restrict your progress and slow down your recovery. Recognize that you may stumble from time to time, but rest assured that you will regain control. The bottom line is that you need to manage your emotions and not be managed by them. As you learn to accept reality and change what you can, you will find that these emotions will not reach crisis proportions, and with each success, you will find yourself in greater control.

### BETH'S PERSPECTIVE

Beth told us how hard it was to adjust to living with heart disease:

> I was so angry and scared when I had my heart attack that I spent most of my time silently fuming and withdrawing from my family. I had exercised all my life and thought I was doing everything I could to be healthy, to no avail. I soon realized, however, that I wasn't helping myself or others by sulking and holding all my emotions back. So I got help. I began talking to my family and my doctor. I entered a cardiac rehab program where I met others who were just as angry and scared as I was. I still have bouts of anger and anxiety, but I deal with them one step at a time, and I'm slowly becoming more confident in my abilities. If I have one piece of advice to give, it would be to have faith in yourself and get help when you need it.

## How to Get Help

The impact of being diagnosed with heart disease may result in an overwhelming feeling of helplessness or loss of control. This will affect your ability to clearly make decisions about your job, your family, or other issues that may arise. For others, adjusting to a new lifestyle can be extremely difficult. If these problems occur, individual counseling may be beneficial. Seek help from your doctor or a trained counselor.

---

**CALMING YOUR FEARS:**
**TAKE CHARGE OF YOUR EMOTIONS**

- Coping with the emotional impact of illness can be longer lasting than the physical impact of illness. Unknowns and uncertainties leave you feeling vulnerable about your health, your family, and your job.
- Common emotional responses to illness include: denial, anxiety, fear of death, loss of confidence, anger, and depression. When left unmanaged, some of these emotions may lead to an exaggeration of your illness. Learn to confront these emotions in your own way! Don't be afraid to reach out for help.

---

## FAMILY CONCERNS

Your illness will affect your family, but positive changes can result from this experience. During the first days of hospitalization, families commonly learn the details of the physical problem, the medical procedures, and the physical healing, but often do not receive counseling on coping with the emotional issues you will face. This section is devoted to easing that burden and transition. We will discuss how you might expect yourself and loved ones to be affected by your illness and how everyone can learn to heal together.

## Your Role

You may perceive that your role in the family is changing. For example, you may feel that you can't take care of matters for which your family depends on you. Maybe you can't immediately, but this may change at a later date.

Sometimes your family can get lost during your transition. Everything is suddenly different for you, which means that everything is also suddenly different for them, too. It is helpful for you to understand how your family members try to compensate for your feelings of grief and helplessness, but you should also keep in mind that they are not responsible for your health and your health-conscious behavior choices. You are!

## Your Partner

Partners may experience many of the same emotions you do—sadness, anger, fear, depression, and confusion. Your partner may feel a need to have a different relationship with you. He or she may want to protect you from stress or anger and may want to take primary responsibility for finances, child rearing, and managing the home. You may not know how your partner feels because he or she may hide his or her true feelings. Your partner may want to be strong for you and appear in complete control. Keeping up with these challenges, however, can quickly become overwhelming and exhausting, even for a "superperson." After a while, partners may find themselves feeling resentful, having been displaced from their previous comfortable roles.

There are several things that can be done to keep the lines of communication open:

- Discuss feelings openly.
- Identify and discuss new roles. Look for positive ways to make life easier for everyone.
- Discuss how each family member can continue contributing in his/her own way.
- Discuss any limitations and how you think they might be best handled.
- Make healthy living a family affair; for example, grocery shopping, exercising, and cooking together.

In the midst of all of this, partners often forget to care for themselves. Partners need to make sure that they have time to do the things they enjoy, to relax, and to rest. This will help to keep some individual identity and provide stress release.

### Partners—Don't Make This Mistake

Although you want to provide your partner with the comfort and support he or she needs, you must also realize that you are not responsible for this person's health, recovery, or well-being. Your partner is! If you overreact and overprotect, you soon will find yourself losing your identity as a partner. You'll feel more like a nurse than a mate or friend. Your partner likely will lose his or her identity as well. Your job is to support independence, not dependence. Your partner needs to function normally to improve his or her confidence, self-esteem, and ultimately health.

As a couple, you will recover from this experience by realizing that this is not a black-and-white process. Keeping the lines of communication open and supporting one another will make your relationship stronger. Recovery begins with realizing: you need to heal from this event as much as your partner; let your partner do as much for him/herself as possible; responsibilities should be shared; and caretaking roles must be balanced.

## Your Kids

Whether your children are young or grown, they should be part of this healing process. Your first inclination may be to protect them from this experience. Depending on their age and ability to understand, they should be given information and assistance in comprehending what this means to them. They, too, need to be able to express their feelings in an atmosphere of open communication. Adult children also can be a great source of support to you. Adapted from Wayne Sotile's *Psychosocial Interventions for Cardiopulmonary Rehabilitation*, the following eight guidelines for discussing illness with children can be applied with other family members as well. They include advice on making communication age appropriate.

1. Talk about the illness. Begin by talking with your children about how you are reacting to your own fears and frustrations. Giving them a glimpse of how you are thinking about, feeling, and coping with this illness will help children feel more normal and will model for them how they, too, might cope.

2. Ask if they have questions. Find out if they are worrying about what is happening or what will happen now that your family is dealing with your illness.

3. If they have no questions, give them information anyway. Children often listen more than they let you know. Give them information that is appropriate to their age and that conveys hope and confidence that your family will successfully weather this chapter of your life.

4. It's okay to admit that you don't have all the answers. Pretending to know everything just serves to confuse children. Sometimes, the best answer is, "That's a good question. But none of us knows the answer for sure."

5. At the same time, offer reassurance. It is especially important to reassure your children that you are receiving good medical care and that you will continue to do all you can to recover. A good

way to do this is to arrange for them to see you going through your rehabilitation routine. If possible, just seeing how strong and hardy you are can soothe many of your children's fears.

6. Give your children permission to talk with others about their fears. Teenagers, especially, sometimes find brief counseling helpful in coping with their concerns. If you have only recently had surgery or a medical crisis, inform school guidance counselors to be especially attentive to your children.

7. Emphasize to your children that they had nothing to do with your illness. Children are self-centered in their insecurities, and they need explicit reassurance that their behavior did not cause the illness.

8. Keep communicating! As your rehabilitation progresses, talk openly and frequently about cardiopulmonary rehabilitation being a family affair. In these conversations, be sure to point out what you notice and appreciate about each other.

## Healing Together

Now that you have a clearer picture of the impact your illness has on you and your family, it's time to do something about it! Here are some effective strategies that will help the entire family heal together:

- *Be aware of the issues that may delay everyone's progress.* You may initially feel inadequate and incapable of functioning normally. Family members may overreact and be overprotective.

- *Communicate.* It is extremely important for everyone to understand each other's thoughts and feelings. Talk to each other often. Everyone should share their concerns and feelings openly, honestly, and in a direct manner. Effective communication allows everyone to release suppressed emotions and thoughts, to achieve balance and understanding, to clarify expectations, and to problem solve.

- *Compromise.* Try to establish a give-and-take relationship with everyone involved.
- *Seek spiritual opportunities.* If spirituality is a part of your family, use this as a pillar of support. It will help you to accept what cannot be changed and choose attitudes that will lead toward improved health behavior.
- *Work together.* It is often during periods of crisis that families come together and work cooperatively. Everyone should feel a part of the recovery process. Be supportive of others.
- *Share information.* Information about what caused your illness, what is being done to correct the problem, and how to heal both physically and emotionally should be shared with all family members.
- *Celebrate together.* Celebrate each accomplishment, together!

The loving bond of a family relationship will help you to meet the daily challenges that accompany living with heart disease. Take the time to understand what each family member is going through, know that you are all healing during your recovery, and try to be patient during this period of change. We all have times of emotional instability. Sharing this book with your family and friends is a good beginning to understand how to handle these emotional turmoils and to involve everyone in the recovery process.

## Finding Support for You and Your Family

In addition to the benefits that counseling may provide for the entire family, you may find great comfort by joining a support group, especially during your initial adjustment period. Support groups allow you to meet others who are experiencing similar health problems. Learning how others have successfully progressed through their recovery period can help you to dispel myths or misunderstandings about heart disease and clarify the reality of your situation. Observing the success of others can be a great motivator for you.

## CALMING YOUR FEARS:
### HEALING TOGETHER

- Each family member responds to your illness differently. You may initially feel helpless, inadequate, and dependent. Your job is to assume responsibility for your own health. Your partner may feel a need to have a different relationship with you. Partners may overreact and overprotect. The partner's job is to support independence, not dependence. The children should be given information and assistance in understanding that is age appropriate and be able to express their feelings openly. The children's job is to be a part of the healing process.
- You must do as much for yourself as possible, responsibilities should be shared, and healing must take place together.
- Healing involves understanding what may delay everyone's progress, communicating effectively, compromising, seeking spiritual opportunities, working together, sharing information, and celebrating each success!

The physical healing associated with heart disease is usually complete within a relatively short period of time, but the emotional healing can take longer, particularly if feelings are left unmanaged. The time frame for emotional healing will depend on how quickly you and your family can adapt to the reality of your new situation and the change that follows. Each family member should be supportive of others throughout this process. View this time as an opportunity to renew your relationships and gain a sense of security and control.

## RETURNING TO WORK

The decision to return to a full work schedule, to reduce work, or to stop working altogether in order to balance your lifestyle changes should be carefully considered. Don't make any quick judgments. Returning to a meaningful and productive life after being faced with a major health concern involves careful consideration of the physical and mental demands of your job, your ability to meet those demands, your careful assessment of your options, and a review of your life goals and priorities. Others can help you in this process. Your doctor can evaluate your capabilities and limitations and provide specific instructions for you. Your employer can make simple adjustments or job modifications to help make your job more suitable for you, and your family may provide the support, understanding, and patience that you need to discuss possible changes in work roles.

Returning to work can be a therapeutic part of your recovery process. Your self-confidence may improve, your anxiety may lessen, and you may feel reassured that you can live a normal and productive life with heart disease. Advancements in medical technology and pharmaceutical breakthroughs have led to a trend toward an earlier return to work following a cardiac event. Today, most people are able to return to work within two to three months after a cardiac event. The average recovery period after a heart attack or coronary artery bypass surgery is approximately six to twelve weeks, and possibly less after angioplasty (PTCA).

This section will help to get you prepared to return to work. We will discuss the "Getting Ready" period that involves preparing yourself for the physical and mental demands of work, the "Getting Set" period that involves learning your strengths, your limitations, and your options early on so that you can make an informed decision about returning to work, and the "Go" period that involves learning what to expect before you go back and what to watch out for to prevent health setbacks.

## Get Ready

You may be anxious about returning to work, but you need not be. Tell yourself you can do it—one step at a time. Your first step should be to focus on getting your strength back and getting yourself in the right frame of mind. Rest assured that as you improve in these areas, you will find that your motivation and confidence improve. Allow yourself time to mend physically and mentally.

### *Getting Your Strength Back*

The physical preparation required for you to return to work is similar to the physical training required to improve the function of your heart. We will discuss the best strategies for designing an exercise program that is safe, enjoyable, and well-suited to your needs in chapter 4. In addition to your regular exercise program, your doctor may suggest a specific weight-training program if your job requires some form of manual labor.

Exercise has many health benefits, including improved strength, stamina, and endurance. This will help you to return to work. As you begin your regular exercise program, keep in mind that it takes approximately eight to twelve weeks to improve your fitness level, and regular participation in physical activity thereafter to maintain improved fitness.

If you return to work before you have become properly conditioned, you may find that you tire more easily and do not have the strength or stamina required for your work schedule. Don't panic. This does not mean that you have to stop working altogether. It simply is an indication that you need to make some minor adjustments until you are feeling stronger.

Some people who return to work early find that a gradual transition from part-time to full-time employment is best. Begin part-time and gradually add hours as you feel ready. If you find that you are consistently fatigued at the end of each day, you are probably pushing yourself too hard and you should ease off by lightening your workload or the amount of time spent on the job. Transition gradually to your desired number of work hours.

### *The Right Frame of Mind*

The next step should be to prepare yourself mentally for the challenges of work demands and the mental stresses that await you. Establishing the right frame of mind can help you to meet these challenges and ease your transition back to work. The psychological impact of being diagnosed with heart disease can impair your confidence, your motivation, your ability to make decisions, your judgment, and your relationships with other people. Emotional distress (feelings of anger, frustration, anxiety, depression, and fear) also can slow your recovery process and decrease your confidence about your ability to return to work.

Your psychological recovery begins with your evaluation of these feelings. Talk to someone about your concerns and where you think you are in the process of recovery. Be patient. Taking charge of your emotions is not easy; a gradual approach works best. Handling the impact of being diagnosed with heart disease and regaining your confidence, motivation, judgment, decision-making abilities, and relationships with other people, will occur over time and as your physical health improves. Receiving supportive feedback from others and practicing stress management techniques regularly (see chapter 6) may help lessen your emotional distress and aid in your speedy psychological recovery.

If you find you are not progressing as fast as you would like to, you may want to seek help from a trained counselor. A counselor can help you to work through the emotional healing process that follows a life-threatening illness. A counselor also can help you reestablish a positive outlook on life and get you into the right frame of mind for returning to work. Don't overlook the need for mental preparation for returning to work. Mental healing is as important as physical healing and is often the determining factor in your successful return to work.

**BRAD'S PERSPECTIVE**

Brad is a patient who survived a cardiac arrest. Here's what he had to say about how he prepared himself physically and mentally to return to work:

> I participated in a cardiac rehabilitation program for twelve weeks at a hospital nearby. While there, I learned how to exercise and adjust my diet. I felt better after I began exercising regularly and soon found myself supplementing my cardiac rehab exercise program at home. Through exercise, I also gained confidence that I could handle work conditions and the stress of work better. My outlook improved even more when I read about other people who had the same experiences. But, I have to admit, my doctor helped me too. She showed a genuine concern for my condition and gave me the encouragement I needed to lead a normal life again.

## Get Set

Getting set involves learning your strengths, your limitations, and your options early on so that you can make an informed decision about returning to work. Have an open discussion with your doctor about this issue. Be honest about your concerns and fears. Your doctor will want to know details about what type of work you do and your work environment. Together you can develop a plan of action for your return to work. It is important for you to be open about these details with your doctor so that he or she can plan the best possible strategy for your safe return.

### *What Are My Limitations?*

Your doctor may have you complete an exercise stress test to determine your ability to tolerate physical activity. A stress test identifies your maximum physical activity tolerance and can be compared to the amount of energy required to do your specific job to determine if your current job is safe for you. Energy to tolerate physical activity and to perform your job can be expressed in terms of METS, an abbreviation for metabolic equivalent. One MET, for example, is equivalent to the amount of energy you consume at rest (3.5 ml of oxygen/kilogram of body weight each minute). Table 3.1 lists common MET equivalents ranging from 1 to 10+ for various home, work, and recreational activities. Use this chart to get a feel for how your doctor determines safe activities for you based on your current health status.

For example, if your maximum physical activity tolerance is 7 METS, your doctor may advise home and occupational activities that do not exceed this energy equivalent.

Be careful when using this information. It serves as a guide to knowing the types of activities you may safely perform. However, factors such as fatigue, emotional distress, excitement, and your level of fitness can change a MET level for any given activity.

Learning about your physical limitations is important and can give you confidence about what activities you can safely perform. As you become more physically fit, you will be able to do more without becoming tired. This will become evident on a follow-up stress test or performing at the same MET level without symptoms such as shortness of breath or chest pain. This is a great confidence booster and something to look forward to! Making improvements, both physically and mentally, can ease your transition back to work and back to your normal daily living activities.

Once you learn the specifics about what activities you can do safely, you will be instructed to return to work without limitations, to return to work with limitations, or to not return to work at all. Take the time to carefully consider all your options.

**TABLE 3.1     Determining Safe Activity Levels**

Use this chart as a reference for relating MET measurements to energy costs of various home, exercise, and work activities. Remember, this chart is only meant to provide you with a general reference point. Confirm with your doctor your safe activity levels.

| METS | HOME ACTIVITIES | WORK/EXERCISE ACTIVITIES |
|------|-----------------|--------------------------|
| 1 | Resting, sitting, eating, reading, bed rest, sewing, watching TV. | Work/exercise activities do not apply. |
| 1–2 | Dressing, shaving, bathing, brushing teeth, making bed, knitting, card playing, standing. | Word processing, desk work, driving car, walking 1 mph on level ground. |
| 2–3 | Cooking, tub bathing, waxing floor, playing piano, light woodworking. | Riding power lawn mower, using hand tools, janitoral work, repairing car, walking 2 mph on level ground, bicycling 5 mph, playing billiards, fishing, bowling, golfing (using cart), operating a motorboat, horseback riding (slowly). |
| 3–4 | General housework, light gardening, cleaning windows, pushing light power mower, using wheelbarrow for 100-pound load, sexual intercourse. | Driving large truck, welding, bricklaying, plastering, assembly-line work, walking 3 mph, bicycling 6 mph, sailing (small boat), golfing (using hand cart), horseshoes, fly-fishing (waders), archery, badminton (doubles), horseback riding (at slow trot), playing music energetically. |

*continued on next page*

TABLE 3.1    *continued*

| METS | HOME ACTIVITIES | WORK/EXERCISE ACTIVITIES |
|---|---|---|
| 4–5 | Heavy housework, heavy gardening, light home repairs, raking leaves, hoeing. | Painting, masonry, paper-hanging, calisthenics, table tennis, golfing (carrying bag), tennis (doubles), dancing, slow swimming, walking 3.5 mph, bicycling 8 mph, fox-trot dancing. |
| 5–6 | Digging in garden, shoveling light loads. | Sawing softwood, using heavy tools, lifting 50 pounds, walking 4 mph, bicycling 10 mph, ice/roller skating, fishing with waders, hiking, hunting, canoeing 4 mph, horseback riding (posting to trot). |
| 6–7 | Shoveling snow (10 pounds), splitting wood, mowing lawn with hand mower. | All work activities previously listed, walking or jogging at 5 mph, bicycling 11 mph, tennis (singles), waterskiing, light downhill skiing, badminton (competitive), square dancing. |
| 7–8 | Moving heavy furniture. | Sawing hardwood, digging ditches, lifting 80 pounds, paddleball, touch football, swimming (backstroke), basketball, ice hockey, running 5 mph, horseback riding (gallop), mountain climbing. |

**TABLE 3.1**    *continued*

| METS | HOME ACTIVITIES | WORK/EXERCISE ACTIVITIES |
|---|---|---|
| 8–9 | Shoveling (14 pounds). | Lifting 100 pounds, running 5.5 mph, bicycling 13 mph, swimming (breaststroke), handball (social), cross-country skiing, fencing, squash (social). |
| 10+ | Shoveling (16 pounds). | Running 6 mph or faster, handball (competitive), squash (competitive), gymnastics, football (contact). |

*Source: Adapted from S. M. Fox, J. P. Naughton, and P. A. Gorman, "Physical Activity and Cardiovascular Health. III. The Exercise Prescription; frequency and type of activity."* Modern Concepts of Cardiovascular Disease *41, no. 6 (1972).*

### Consider Your Options

When your work requirements exceed your ability to perform them, you have several options from which to choose:

1. Modify your job. To make your job more suitable, it may be modified by a change in your job duties or a change in the environment in which you are expected to perform these duties. These changes often involve simple adjustments and are made by your employer after careful consideration of the nature of your work, work policies, and your doctor's recommendations. Modifying your job involves a collaborative effort between you and your employer. Have an open discussion with your employer about your current and long-term limitations. Together you can set the pace for getting back to work.

2. Seek an alternative job. In some cases, where the work demands of your position cannot be altered, you may be placed in a completely different job that is better suited for you. Sometimes this can be with the same employer and other times this is not feasible. Some form of vocational training may be helpful in either case.

3. Consider the benefits of vocational training. In addition to the recommendations of your doctor, a vocational counselor can evaluate your job in relation to your health status and assist you with the behavioral aspects of your recovery. The counselor can provide you with guidance in returning to your present job, a new perspective on alternative job choices, insights into making changes in your duties at your present job, and a better understanding of the emotional, social, and financial adaptations that may be necessary during your recovery period and quite possibly when you are well again.

4. Get help from others. In addition to the benefits that may be gained by vocational counseling, support groups may provide additional assistance in this area (see appendix A).

5. Improve your physical capacity. Participating in a regular exercise program will enhance your endurance. Find out if your nearby hospital offers a cardiac rehabilitation program.

6. Have an open discussion with your doctor. Find out if there is another treatment available that may stabilize your clinical condition so that you are able to tolerate higher levels of activity and exercise training.

7. Seek psychological and emotional support from others. Your doctor, your counselor, your family, your friends, your neighbors, and your clergy all may assist you with making decisions about your job. You don't have to go it alone.

8. Quit work. You may find that work is not the best option for you at the present time due to the physical or emotional demands of your job. You may wish to seek counseling to help

you with your transition out of the workforce. Vocational counselors are helpful in this area. If you find that work is not a viable option for you, consider the alternatives: qualifying for Social Security disability insurance or retirement status. If factors such as the degree of your disability and your medical prognosis prohibit your return to work for a period of at least one year, you may apply for Social Security Disability Insurance. This can be done by simply completing an application at a Social Security office near you. You are also eligible to receive vocational services, which are provided by each state.

Your doctor's and employer's recommendations are important and will influence in what capacity you will return to work. You should also be an active participant in this discussion. Talk to your personnel office regarding your legal rights. Work should provide you with a certain level of satisfaction and economic security. Negotiate your options where possible and make the best use of your abilities.

### BRAD'S PERSPECTIVE

Brad returned to work for about three months but decided to retire after that. Here's what he had to say:

Although I felt healthy and able to work, I discovered that work wasn't fun anymore. I knew I could do it if I wanted, but I guess I discovered more important things in life. I was in a position to retire so I did just that! After being retired for seven years I decided to go to work at a garden center on a part-time basis. It has its ups and downs, but I really enjoy the work and interaction with others.

## Go!

Are you ready? Once you have gotten the green light to return to work, it is helpful to know what to expect in terms of physical and emotional responses. Additionally, you may find that learning to cope with the challenges of work-related stress will help you to strike a healthy balance between work demands and time for relaxation.

### *Know What to Expect*

Returning to work will be different. You are no longer the same person. You have changed as a result of coming face to face with a life-threatening illness. Here is what you can expect when you return to work:

- You may feel overwhelmed at first. All of your colleagues will want to know how you are doing as soon as you see them. Some may treat you differently because they don't understand your illness. Decide how much information about your illness you want to share with your co-workers before returning. You may find it helpful to let them know how well you feel.

- The pace may seem quicker than it did before. Don't try to take on too much too soon. Talk to your employer about pacing yourself and easing back into your routines.

- You may find that some of your old work habits will need to be changed. You might consider making some changes in your daily routine to include periodic rest breaks. You may be surprised at how a rest break can help you feel refreshed and ready to take on your next assignment.

- You may feel awkward about taking your medications at work. If you feel this way, look for a private place to do this.

- You will want to control your job-related stress more than ever. Try to adopt some of the coping strategies outlined in chapter 6 and practice them at work on a regular basis. Taking a moment to take a breather, daydream, or stretch your muscles may help to put you in a better frame of mind.

- It is not uncommon to struggle with negative emotions when you first return to work, especially if you are not able to do as much at work as you once could. Remember, counseling may help you to mentally prepare for and transition back to work successfully.
- You may feel as though you should return to a full work schedule. Do you eventually want to do so? Carefully consider your options. Is working part-time a possibility? Could you work periodically at home?
- You may discover a need to investigate other career options. Explore them! Learning about your alternatives is great, but try not to burden yourself with a quick change.

### SUSAN'S PERSPECTIVE

Susan, who had heart valve replacement surgery, has some advice on returning to work as well:

My advice on returning to work is to maintain positive thoughts, actively participate in a cardiac rehab program, supplement your rehab program with additional exercise, watch your diet, and participate in other activities such as gardening, volunteer work, working around home, and traveling. Doing the things you enjoy will give you a sense of satisfaction in your life and will help you to be happy at work.

## *Watch for Signs of Trouble*

In some cases, the first signs of trouble may be a mismatch between the physical or emotional requirements of your job and what you are able to currently handle. Sometimes, you may not realize this problem until you are "back in the saddle" again. In other cases, the first signs of trouble may be seen by a change in your health. In either case, be on the lookout for these signs of trouble and report these symptoms to your doctor immediately if they occur:

- Increasing levels of fatigue on a regular basis after work.
- Experiencing symptoms at work such as angina, shortness of breath, dizziness, or fatigue.
- Taking increased amounts of medication to function at work.

**CALMING YOUR FEARS:**
**RETURNING TO WORK**

- *Get Ready:* Prepare yourself mentally and physically so that you can meet the everyday challenges of your workday.
- *Get Set:* Learn your strengths, your limitations, and your options early on so that you can make informed decisions.
- *Go:* Know what to expect before you return to work, and learn the signs to watch for to prevent complications from occurring. Learn to cope with the challenges of work-related stress (see chapter 6 for more details).

## INTIMACY

People who are diagnosed with heart disease are usually able to resume most of their activities. This includes sexual intimacy. Using common sense and following a few basic guidelines can enable a return to the most special function of the heart, the act of loving.

### The Act of Loving

As a general rule, if you are able to climb two flights of steps without experiencing shortness of breath, chest pain, or fatigue, you are ready to resume sexual relations. A more scientific evaluation of your readiness to resume sexual relations can be determined by your doctor after you complete a stress test. Normal physical reactions to sex are a moist, warm flushed skin or heightened skin color and a slight increase in breathing. These are not signs of heart strain.

### Read On, You Sexy Devil

The cardiac risks of sex are far less than you might expect. People who have had a heart attack often resume their previous sex lives within four to eight weeks after the attack. People who have had heart surgery often resume sexual relationships within one to three weeks after hospital discharge. Don't try to do too much too quickly, but don't be so fearful that you don't try at all. If you have been following your doctor's orders and have begun exercising, then you are likely ready to resume sexual relations.

Keep in mind that exercise strengthens the heart and lets the heart perform the same amount of work with less stress. Exercise also makes you feel more confident in what your body can do. It is a good way to prepare yourself to return to your daily activities, including sexual relations. As your physical condition improves, you also may find that you tolerate sexual relations better, have fewer symptoms, and find your sexual relations more enjoyable.

## Setting the Mood

The following practices may increase your emotional satisfaction while at the same time reduce the likelihood that physical or emotional problems may arise during sex:

- *Communication.* Discuss and share with your partner your feelings, fears, and anxieties about resuming sexual activity. Having heart disease can be very stressful for you and your family. Do not put unrealistic performance goals on you and your partner. Be aware that your partner may become overprotective of you.
- *Usual partner.* Sex should be with your usual partner. Sex with new partners requires more energy and puts more stress on your heart.
- *Medications.* Some medications may cause a decrease in sex drive or function. Ask your doctor if you think your medications may be causing a problem for you.
- *Getting in touch.* Sharing hugs and backrubs are warm ways to get back in touch with your sexual partner.
- *Position.* No major changes in your usual sexual position are necessary. For eight weeks after open-heart surgery, use positions that do not require supporting your weight on your arms.
- *Foreplay.* Begin with sexual foreplay. This allows for a gradual increase in heart rate and blood pressure.
- *Masturbation.* Masturbation helps some people regain self-confidence in their sexuality. It may also ease the transition to intercourse, since it expends less of the body's energy.
- *Oral-genital sex.* Oral-genital sex places no undue stress on the heart. However, anal intercourse may lead to irregular heart rhythms and should be discussed with your doctor first.
- *Extramarital affairs.* Extramarital affairs should be avoided because they usually result in heightened emotional stress. Less than 1 percent of deaths from a heart attack are related to sexual activity, but most of these deaths occurred during extramarital affairs.

- *Smoking.* If you choose to continue smoking, do not smoke one hour before sex.
- *Atmosphere.* Have sex in pleasant surroundings. Avoid extremes in temperature.
- *Eating.* Wait at least three hours after eating heavy foods or drinking alcohol before engaging in sexual activity.
- *Nitroglycerin.* Your doctor may prescribe taking nitroglycerin before sex to prevent chest pain from occurring during relations.
- *Angina.* Angina may result from sexual intercourse, just as it may from other forms of exertion. If angina occurs during sex, stop your activity for a while. Take nitroglycerin as directed by your doctor and rest.

## A COUPLE'S PERSPECTIVE

Martha's husband James had coronary artery bypass surgery two years ago. Here is what they told us about how they've handled sexual intimacy:

*James:* It's funny, really. I think Martha's and my physical relationship is almost better than it was before my surgery. Once I realized I wasn't going to die, I began to relax and not put pressure on myself to perform. We spend much more time with foreplay, take baths together, and cuddle in front of the fireplace.

*Martha:* It was scary at first. I spent the first few months afraid to let him touch me. I wanted to satisfy him and not have him overexert himself trying to satisfy me. We talked about my fears and his anxiety, and now we just take it slowly with no expectation. In many ways we are more intimate than we were before; coming so close to death has really made us value just being close.

## Difficulties in Resuming Sexual Relations

Some people report difficulties in resuming sexual relations for a number of reasons: fear of chest pain, fear of death, fear of sexual dysfunction, and fear of another heart attack. Don't get discouraged! You can calm these fears quickly by talking with your doctor or a trained counselor. These experts can help you to reestablish your relationship with your partner, overcome sexual dysfunction, adjust to changing sexual patterns, understand the risks of sexual intercourse, and conquer your fears. Don't avoid returning to your full level of sexual functioning because you are afraid to do so! Get answers to your questions now. Learning the best time to resume sexual relations and what your limitations are will help to decrease feelings of fear and uncertainty.

### CALMING YOUR FEARS:
#### RESUMING SEXUAL RELATIONS

- Climbing two flights of stairs comfortably is one indication of your readiness to resume sexual relations. Check with your doctor to be sure that this activity is safe for you.
- Certain sexual practices may decrease physical and emotional problems and may increase satisfaction. Review the section on "Setting the Mood."
- Difficulties in resuming sexual relations are common and are often related to fear. Seeking help from qualified professionals may help you to reestablish your relationship with your partner, overcome sexual dysfunction, adjust to changing sexual patterns, understand the risks of sexual intercourse, and improve your confidence!

## THE NEW YOU

Coping with illness is not easy. Beyond the physical healing that takes place, you need to heal emotionally as well. Understand that there are normal emotional responses to a health crisis: denial, anxiety, fear of death, loss of confidence, anger, and depression. When left unresolved, these emotional responses can quickly sap your energy and restrict your progress. Don't let them! Remember, improvements in your ability and your independence will help you to gain control over these emotional responses. Seeking assistance from others and involving family members in the healing process also will help in easing the impact of your emotional reactions.

Lifestyle adjustments reach far beyond simply dealing with emotional issues, return-to-work issues, and intimacy considerations. The challenge of your recovery involves establishing priorities and goals that will allow you to grab hold of what is important to you in life. Goals that include physical, spiritual, mental, social, and emotional components will likely contribute to your speedy return to good health. The restrictions on lifestyle once associated with heart disease (limited physical exertion, no lifting arms above your head, no driving, not returning to work, no sexual relations) have long been dispensed with, so set your mind at ease. You can return to an active, fulfilling life.

&

## CHAPTER FOUR

# GETTING COMFORTABLE WITH EXERCISE

REGULAR EXERCISE IS AN IMPORTANT STEP ON YOUR JOURNEY toward good health. You will feel good, you will look good, and your outlook for the future will improve. Your primary exercise training goal will be to strengthen your heart so that you can continue to live an active, healthy life.

Exercising regularly is one of the best gifts you can give yourself. It improves the function of your heart, strengthens your muscles, helps to lower your blood pressure, controls your cholesterol levels, and aids in weight reduction. It also will help your medication to work effectively, and it can lessen symptoms of shortness of breath, chest pain, and fatigue.

This chapter will guide you in the process of establishing an exercise program that is safe, enjoyable, and suited to your needs. You will learn what type of exercise is best, and how often, how hard, and how long you should exercise at each session. You will also learn to identify warning signs that tell you to either adjust your exercise program or call your doctor for advice.

## YOUR EXERCISE PROGRAM

It is important to consider your specific medical history, so that you can design a program that meets your health needs, ability level, and goals. You should start slowly, progress gradually, and maintain safety at all times. With this in mind, you can create a program to achieve your health and fitness goals. Before you begin, consult your doctor for exercise guidelines.

Your exercise program will include three essential parts: 1) warm-up, 2) conditioning, and 3) cool-down. Each phase of your exercise program is necessary and allows the body to safely adapt to the changes it undergoes during exercise. Following this specific exercise plan will help you to improve your fitness level within eight to twelve weeks.

### A NOTE TO FAMILY AND FRIENDS

You can get involved too! Exercise can serve a dual purpose: when you exercise along with your loved one you help motivate him or her, as well as take good care of your own health. You, too, can use this chapter as a resource to get you started and keep you moving. Exercising together is a good way to monitor your loved one's progress and improve your confidence that he or she is on the road to recovery.

## The Warm-Up Phase

The warm-up phase of exercise gradually prepares your body for more strenuous activity by increasing circulation to all muscles used. This phase consists of low-level endurance activities followed by stretching. Low-level activities prepare you for more vigorous aerobic exercise by increasing the blood flow to your muscles.

Examples of this type of exercise include range of motion activities (for example, repetitive arm or leg movements), slow walking, or using light tension on a piece of exercise equipment.

Stretching prepares your muscles for activity, loosens your joints, relieves muscle tension, and improves the body's ability to move freely. To guide you in the process of stretching, we have included easy-to-follow examples at the end of this chapter. When stretching, avoid bouncing or jerking-type movements as they may force your muscles beyond their maximum ranges, thus increasing your risk of injury. It is also important to exhale while going into a stretch, to hold the stretch for a period of approximately fifteen to twenty seconds, and to breathe normally throughout the stretch.

You should spend a minimum of five to ten minutes on warm-up activities and stretching. Completing this part of your exercise program will decrease the likelihood of problems during the next phase. Once you have finished your warm-up, you are ready for conditioning.

## The Conditioning Phase

The conditioning phase of the exercise program is where the desired training effect takes place. To design your individualized exercise plan, you will need to outline what kind of exercise you intend to do (type), how many days a week you will exercise (frequency), the length of time you will devote to exercise each session (duration), and how much effort you should put forth while exercising (intensity). Learning to balance each of these parts will help you to achieve and maintain a higher level of physical fitness and improve the function of your heart. Don't worry if you're not comfortable exercising yet—we'll be with you every step of the way.

### Exercise Type

Aerobic exercise is the preferred type of activity for improving the function of your heart because it allows the lungs and heart to take in and distribute oxygen efficiently to all parts of the body. It also increases your muscles' ability to power your movement. There are long-lasting benefits of aerobic exercise. Improvements in fitness will decrease the demands on your heart and reduce your fatigue, letting you perform normal daily activities with plenty of energy left over.

Examples of aerobic exercise include brisk walking, rowing, cycling (stationary or outdoor), swimming, various types and levels of aerobic dancing, jogging, stair-stepping, and simulated cross-country skiing. One is not particularly better than another, but those that allow your arms and legs to work together are preferred. Choose activities that you will enjoy and that you will perform on a regular basis. This will help you to stay motivated.

### Exercise Frequency

Exercise should be performed on a regular basis at least three days per week. If you are a beginner and/or if you have any limitations, choose to exercise on alternate days to allow for adequate amounts of rest in between each exercise session. As you gradually progress in your program, the frequency can be increased from three days to as many as five days per week depending on your interests, goals, and recommendations from your doctor.

Getting more than five days of aerobic exercise per week is generally not recommended, since it will cause muscle fatigue and increase your risk of injury. On the other hand, inconsistent effort (fewer than three days per week) will limit your progress. Your exercise frequency should always meet the minimum requirements so that you can achieve the health benefits associated with activity. Try to maintain regularity with your exercise program at all times.

### Exercise Duration

The length of the exercise session, excluding the warm-up and the cool-down, is the duration. There is no standard exercise duration recommendation for all individuals. The duration of your exercise should be gradually increased from as little as five minutes of exercise (for beginners) to as much as twenty to forty-five minutes (for more advanced individuals). How long you should exercise at first will depend on several factors: 1) how long you were ill; 2) how active or inactive you have been; and 3) how healthy you are right now. If, for example, it's hard for you to exercise for ten minutes, try two periods of five minutes each with two-minute breaks in between. Then build from there. You will eventually achieve the fitness goal of continuous exercise for twenty to forty-five minutes.

### Exercise Intensity

Your exercise intensity level should always feel comfortable, yet be strenuous enough so that you feel challenged. There are ways to regulate your exercise intensity. The best way to maintain the correct level is to monitor your heart rate while you are exercising, pay attention to how you feel during exercise, and notice your ability to talk during exercise.

### Monitoring Your Heart Rate

Monitoring your heart rate during exercise involves learning what your heart rate should be and learning how to check your pulse during exercise. Your heart rate is the number of times your heart beats in one minute. At rest, your heart typically beats about 60 to 90 times per minute. During exercise, however, your heart rate will increase beyond this resting level. How much it increases depends on how hard you are exercising. The harder you work, the higher your heart rate will climb.

Your target heart rate represents how fast your heart should beat during exercise (for example, 110 to 140 beats/minute). These boundaries let you work hard enough to condition your heart and muscles, yet not so hard that you place undue stress on your heart. During the early stages of your exercise program, you may wish to exercise below your target heart rate until your levels of strength, stamina, and endurance improve. As you progress and your fitness level grows, your goal should be to consistently exercise within this heart rate range. Exercising above your target heart rate is not recommended. This can place undue stress on the heart and gives no additional fitness benefits. Your doctor should recommend a target heart rate based on your most recent stress test, your medications, and your medical history.

You can approximate your target heart rate range by using a simple formula. Use Table 4.1 to find your target heart rate range. You will need to know 1) how to determine your maximal heart rate, 2) how to determine your conditioning intensity, and 3) how to check your pulse. Your maximal heart rate is your highest heart rate achieved at the end of your exercise stress test. If you do not know what this exact number is, ask your doctor. You can also estimate your maximal heart rate by using a simple formula:

220 – your age = estimated maximal heart rate

General recommendations for determining your conditioning intensity include using a range from 50 percent for your lower limit to 85 percent for your upper limit. Use the example in Table 4.1 as a point of reference for determining your estimated target heart rate range. Refer to the section on checking your heart rate later in this chapter to learn how to determine your resting heart rate.

With this information, you can fill in the blank spaces on Table 4.1 to obtain the lower and upper limits of your estimated target heart rate range. Keep in mind that this approximated target heart rate may vary as a result of any changes in your medical condition or medications, and with the results of new exercise stress tests.

Table 4.2 shows estimated target heart rates for different age categories prepared by the American Heart Association. To use this table, look for the age category closest to yours and read across to find your target heart rate. Remember, these figures are averages and should be used as general guidelines.

**TABLE 4.1    How to Calculate Your Target Heart Rate**

| | LOWER LIMIT (Example) | CALCULATE YOUR LOWER LIMIT HERE | UPPER LIMIT (Example) | CALCULATE YOUR UPPER LIMIT HERE |
|---|---|---|---|---|
| Maximal Heart Rate* | 180 | | 180 | |
| Resting Heart Rate: | − 60 | | − 60 | |
| | 120 | | 120 | |
| Conditioning Intensity: | x .50 | | x .85 | |
| | 60 | | 102 | |
| Resting Heart Rate: | + 60 | | + 60 | |
| | 120 | | 162 | |
| Target Heart Rate: | 120 (Your Lower Limit) | | 162 (Your Upper Limit) | |

*Individual Maximal Heart Rate varies. Your medical history, current medications, exercise history, and physical condition will influence this number. This formula should not be used as a substitute for your doctor's recommendations. Confirm with your doctor that this calculated target heart rate is suitable for you before beginning your exercise program.

TABLE 4.2      **Estimated Target Heart Rates**

| AGE (YEARS) | HEART RATE ZONE (50–75%) | AVERAGE MAXIMUM HEART RATE (100%) |
|---|---|---|
| 20 years | 100–150 beats per minute | 200 |
| 25 years | 98–146 beats per minute | 195 |
| 30 years | 95–143 beats per minute | 190 |
| 35 years | 93–139 beats per minute | 185 |
| 40 years | 90–135 beats per minute | 180 |
| 45 years | 88–131 beats per minute | 175 |
| 50 years | 85–128 beats per minute | 170 |
| 55 years | 83–124 beats per minute | 165 |
| 60 years | 80–120 beats per minute | 160 |
| 65 years | 78–116 beats per minute | 155 |
| 70 years | 75–113 beats per minute | 150 |

*Source: American Heart Association World Wide Web Site,* Heart and Stroke Guide Section, *1996. Copyright © American Heart Association. Reproduced with permission.*

## *A Note of Caution*

There is one exception to the guidelines for estimating your target heart rate. Certain heart medications change your heart rate's response to exercise. An example of this is beta blocker medication, which lowers your resting heart rate and prevents its rise during exercise. If you are taking this type of medicine, the use of the scientific formula for estimating your target heart rate is *not* accurate. General recommendations, in this case, include maintaining an exercise heart rate range that is approximately fifteen to thirty beats above your resting heart rate. Your doctor may recommend a heart rate limit outside of these formulas due to circumstances related to your medical history.

Once you know what your target heart rate is, it will be easier for you to make adjustments to your exercise levels as needed. For example, if your heart rate is below your target while exercising, you may want to increase the intensity of your workout. If, on the other hand, you are exercising above your target heart rate, you should decrease your intensity to keep your heart rate within your target range. You can learn to monitor your heart rate and regulate your exercise intensity by checking your pulse periodically during exercise.

### Checking Your Heart Rate (Pulse)

The words heart rate and pulse mean the same thing. When a health care provider checks your pulse, he or she is checking the number of times your heart beats in one minute. Once you have mastered the technique of pulse taking, you should check it before you exercise, during exercise, after exercise, if you feel dizzy, and if you feel your heart beating irregularly.

Your pulse should be within ten beats of your pre-exercise resting heart rate after you have cooled down from exercise. If it takes longer than ten minutes for your heart rate to return to this level, you probably did not take enough time to adequately cool down. If, on the other hand, you feel dizzy or continue to have a fast heartbeat (above 100) at rest, report your pulse rate and symptoms to your doctor. You can follow these easy steps in Figure 4.1 to learn how to master the technique of pulse checking.

Checking your pulse accurately takes a little patience and a lot of practice. Try not to get discouraged if you have some difficulty at first. Master the technique at rest before you attempt to check it during exercise. If you find that you continue to have difficulty checking your pulse accurately, consider purchasing a pulse meter (a device that automatically registers your pulse and transmits it to a watch). More information about purchasing pulse meters can be found in appendix C.

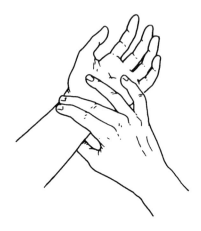

1. Find a watch or clock with a second hand.

2. Place your first two fingers on the thumb side of your wrist.

3. Apply a slight pressure. Do not press too hard.

4. Count your pulse for ten seconds, then multiply by 6 to determine the number of times your heart is beating each minute.

**FIGURE 4.1**    **Pulse Checking**
Illustration by Susan Spellman

### Determining How You Feel

Another method of monitoring your intensity to avoid excess strain while you exercise is to ask yourself how you feel during exercise, using the subjective rating scale in Table 4.3.

Your perception of your exercise intensity should typically fall within the 11 to 14 range on the scale each time you work out. If your level goes beyond 14, you are probably exercising too hard and you should reduce your level of work. Use this commonsense approach to guiding your exercise intensity whenever you feel that you are becoming short of breath or extremely tired.

If you know you have an irregular pulse rate (for example, atrial fibrillation) that your doctor has evaluated, this commonsense method of monitoring your exercise intensity may be particularly useful (especially if you have difficulty in finding and/or counting your pulse rate accurately). Always concentrate on how you are responding throughout your exercise session and expect day-to-day variations in how you feel.

**TABLE 4.3    Perceived Exertion Scale**

| | |
|---|---|
| 6 | |
| 7 | **very, very light** |
| 8 | |
| 9 | **very light** |
| 10 | |
| 11 | **light** |
| 12 | |
| 13 | **somewhat hard** |
| 14 | |
| 15 | **hard** |
| 16 | |
| 17 | **very hard** |
| 18 | |
| 19 | **very, very hard** |
| 20 | |

Source: G. A. Borg. "Psychophysical basis of perceived exertion." Medicine and Science in Sports and Exercise, 14 (1982): 377–381.

*Determining Your Ability to Talk*

During exercise, your rate and depth of breathing should increase but not to a point where you feel extremely short of breath, tired, or uncomfortable. If it is difficult to carry on a conversation with a friend during exercise because you are too short of breath to talk, your exercise intensity level is probably too high and you should reduce it to a more comfortable one. Use the chart in Table 4.4 to help you to know when you should change or stop what you are doing.

**TABLE 4.4    Shortness of Breath Scale**

0 = none

1 = very slight

2 = slight

3 = moderate (think about what you are doing)

4 = somewhat severe (change what you are doing)

5 = severe (stop what you are doing!)

Once the conditioning segment of your exercise program is complete, you should move to your final phase: the cool-down.

## The Cool-Down Phase

The cool-down phase consists of a gradual decrease in your exercise intensity (for example, from a brisk walking pace to a stroll) followed by a series of stretching exercises. Stretching during the cool-down phase helps you to improve flexibility, reduce muscle soreness, and relax. It is during this phase of exercise that your heart rate and blood pressure gradually return to their pre-exercise levels. During both the conditioning and the cool-down phases, exercise should never be stopped abruptly. Stopping abruptly can cause a sudden drop in blood pressure and heart rate, which can cause chest pain, dizziness, and an irregular heart rhythm. Always spend at least five to ten minutes cooling down. Do not hurry to finish.

---

**BOUNCING BACK:**
**YOUR INDIVIDUALIZED EXERCISE PLAN**

*Note:* Check with your doctor before beginning an exercise program.

- *Exercise Type:* Aerobic activities that use the major muscle groups. Examples include brisk walking, cycling, swimming, and aerobic dance. Choose activities that work your arms and legs at the same time.
- *Exercise Frequency:* Start with 3 days per week on alternate days. As you progress, increase to 4–5 days per week as desired.
- *Exercise Duration:* If you tire easily with exercise, start with 2–3 exercise sessions daily of 5–10 minutes each. For the active individual, begin with 12–15 minutes of exercise on alternate days and progress thereafter. Everyone should attempt to progress to a minimum of 30 minutes of exercise.
- *Exercise Intensity:* Exercise within your "target heart rate" every time you work out. Remember that it may take some time to be able to exercise within your target heart rate—be patient. Use a commonsense approach to exercise to determine how you feel. Take the "talk test" each time you exercise with a friend. Consider purchasing a pulse meter if you have difficulty checking your pulse (see appendix C, Selecting an Exercise Program).

## EXERCISE PROGRESSION

You may begin to feel better just a few weeks after starting your new exercise program. You will know you are improving when you are able to do more work at home or when you are exercising with less effort. As you begin to get stronger, you can progress in your exercise program by changing the duration, intensity, and/or type of exercise. How often and by how much you change your program will depend on how well you adapt to each stage.

Plan to increase your exercise program gradually. Progression occurs in three steps:

- *Step 1:* Start off slowly and progress gradually. Start with twelve to fifteen minutes of low-level aerobic activities. If you have difficulty with this, perform multiple exercise bouts of five minutes each, taking two-minute rest breaks in between. Your initial conditioning intensity should fall within a target range of approximately 40 to 60 percent. Exercise three days per week on alternate days. Maintain this pattern for approximately four to six weeks. Take more time if you feel that you are really out of shape (up to or beyond twelve weeks is not uncommon for this stage).
- *Step 2:* Add a few minutes of exercise time every two to three weeks until you can exercise comfortably for twenty to thirty minutes continuously. Your conditioning intensity should fall within a range of approximately 50 to 85 percent. Exercise three to five days per week. Maintain this stage for at least four to five months.
- *Step 3:* At this point, you have reached an exercise level that gives you the health benefits you need. It is no longer necessary to increase exercise time, frequency, and/or intensity. Your goal is to continue with your exercise program on a regular basis to maintain your fitness level. This stage typically begins after six months.

**BOUNCING BACK:**
**THE THREE PHASES OF YOUR EXERCISE PROGRAM**

- *Warm up before you begin* to adequately prepare yourself for exercise. Allow at least 5–10 minutes for low-level endurance activities followed by a series of stretches. Avoid bouncing or jerking-type movements. Do not hold your breath. Hold each stretch 15–20 seconds.
- *Condition yourself gradually.* This is where the desired training effect takes place. There are four parts to improving your fitness level: type, frequency, duration, and intensity of exercise.
- *Cool down after you exercise.* Allow at least 5–10 minutes to perform low-level endurance activities, followed by stretching. Never stop exercise abruptly. Avoid bouncing or jerking-type movements. Do not hold your breath. Hold each stretch 15–20 seconds.

Give yourself at least 8–12 weeks to begin to feel like yourself again.

During each stage of progression, monitor how you feel and your heart rate. Avoid extremely strenuous exercise. The "no pain, no gain" approach will only increase your risk of injury and lessen your interest in the program over time. A slow, systematic approach is both safer and more enjoyable. The more comfortable you are with your exercise program, the more likely you are to stick with it. Copy the exercise record in Figure 4.2 to help you keep track of your exercise program. Share this information with your doctor periodically.

In order to maximize fitness gains while maintaining safety, you

Keep track of your exercise routine by charting your progress below. Share this useful information with your doctor on your next visit.

| DATE | TYPE OF EXERCISE | DURATION | TARGET HEART RATE |
|------|------------------|----------|-------------------|
| 8/15/97 | Walking | 30 minutes | 130–135 beats/minute |

FIGURE 4.2    Sample Exercise Training Record

will need to make periodic adjustments in your exercise program. Recognize that any adjustment you or your doctor make is not a setback. We will discuss later in this chapter the criteria for recognizing the need to alter your exercise program and we will present guidelines for making the appropriate adjustments to your plan.

**BOUNCING BACK:**
**YOUR RATE OF EXERCISE PROGRESSION**

- Start off slowly and progress gradually.
- Follow the three steps of progression: Initial, Improvement, and Maintenance.
- During each stage, monitor how you feel and your heart rate. Avoid strenuous exertion.
- Adjust your program as needed to maintain a comfortable level of exercise at all times.
- You will know you are improving when you are able to do more work at home or when you are exercising with less effort.

## ARE YOU READY TO BEGIN?

Keep in mind a checklist of questions to ask yourself before you begin to exercise. This will help you to make a judgment each day as to whether it is safe for you to exercise. Begin by asking yourself how you feel. Questions should include:

- Have you had any chest pain or shortness of breath today?
- Are you feeling unusually tired?

- Do you have a fever, cold, or the flu?
- Are your ankles or feet swollen? Have you had a weight gain of more than 2 pounds in one day or 5 pounds in one week?
- Are you having trouble sleeping, or did you use more pillows than usual to sleep last night?
- Are you extremely upset today? Did something especially bad happen?
- Did you miss any of your medication today?

If you have answered "yes" to any of these questions, then today is not a good day for you to work out. Exercising when you are sick or emotionally upset puts increased stress on your cardiovascular system that it may not be able to handle. If you exercise without taking your medication, you do not have the protection the medication provides, and you may be prone to chest pain or other problems. If you are already having chest pain or shortness of breath during the day or at night when you are trying to sleep, call your doctor immediately. Do not exercise.

When planning the timing of your exercise session, consider the following issues. You should wait for two hours after consuming a large meal. However, it is important that you do not skip meals. Your body needs fuel to perform at the level required with exercise. A light snack, such as a piece of fruit or crackers before exercise may be helpful. Alcoholic beverages should not be consumed for two hours before and one hour after exercise. Finally, if you continue to smoke, do not smoke for two hours before or one hour after exercise.

Keeping these simple safety tips in mind will ensure a safe exercise session. Remember, most days you will feel good and answer "no" to the questions. And so you are ready to begin to exercise.

## CURRENT VIEWS ON PHYSICAL ACTIVITY

In 1995, the National Institutes of Health published a consensus statement addressing physical activity and cardiovascular health. Its objective was to provide physicians and the general public with an understanding of the relationship between physical activity and cardiovascular health. The conclusions drawn by the panel include the following:

All Americans should engage in regular physical activity at a level appropriate to their capacity, needs, and interest. Children and adults alike should set a goal of accumulating at least thirty minutes of moderate-intensity physical activity on most, and preferably all, days of the week. Most Americans have little or no physical activity in their daily lives, and accumulating evidence indicates that physical inactivity is a major risk factor for cardiovascular disease. However, moderate levels of physical activity confer significant health benefits. Even those who currently meet these daily standards may derive additional health and fitness benefits by becoming more physically active or including more vigorous activity. For those with known cardiovascular disease, cardiac rehabilitation programs that combine physical activity with reduction in other risk factors should be more widely used.

The impetus for this statement was concern that although the mortality rate from cardiovascular disease has declined over the past twenty-five years, heart disease continues to be the leading cause of death. As a population, we are showing improvements in controlling blood pressure, cholesterol, and smoking; however, the risk factors of inactivity and obesity are poorly controlled.

*continued on next page*

**CURRENT VIEWS** *continued*

The statement defines the benefits of physical activity with a goal of achieving thirty minutes of moderate activity daily most and preferably all days of the week. The benefits of moderate-level activity (defined as brisk walking, cycling, swimming, home repair, and yard work), even if performed in ten-minute intervals during the day, will improve overall physical fitness. The statement emphasizes that this is a minimum standard for physical health. People may derive additional health and fitness benefits from becoming even more physically active.

The exercise program presented in this chapter guides you to a level of optimum fitness based on your specific health history. While your exercise program may begin below the minimum standards recommended by the NIH consensus statement, our goal is to help you achieve a level above the minimum standards so that you reap the optimum benefits of exercise. Aerobic exercise at moderate levels as prescribed here will help prevent progression of heart disease and improve control of other risk factors, including high blood pressure, high cholesterol, diabetes, and excess weight.

The NIH consensus statement also encourages individuals who have heart disease to participate in formal cardiac rehabilitation programs that provide education and exercise to prevent progression of the disease. The principles and practices of cardiac rehabilitation programs are the foundation from which this book is written.

## Signals That Your Exercise Intensity Level Is Too High

Avoid the pitfall of trying to do too much too soon with an exercise program. Overexertion will increase your risk of injury, muscle soreness, and other possibly more serious complications. Follow the guidelines for warm-up and cool-down, and exercise time, intensity, and progression. These guidelines will ensure a safe exercise program.

In addition to these guidelines, pay attention to signals from your body that indicate you are doing too much. An easy way to recognize signs of distress is to follow the four P's for exercise safety:

1. *Pain:* If chest, neck, throat, back, or arm discomfort occur during exercise, slow down and stop. Sit down and rest. If the discomfort continues, take one nitroglycerin (NTG) tablet every five minutes until the discomfort is completely gone. If the discomfort is still present after three NTG tablets, call 911 and go to the emergency room. Do not continue taking NTG tablets and do not drive yourself.

2. *Panting:* If you become short of breath to the point that talking becomes very difficult, reduce your work or pace to where you can talk easily.

3. *Perspiration:* It is normal to perspire during exercise; however, a chilled feeling accompanied by cold and moist skin could be a sign of an abnormal response to activity. If this occurs, reduce your work or pace.

4. *Pulse:* If you are above your target heart rate, reduce the work or pace so that you are within the target heart rate.

Dizziness is not a normal response to exercise. If dizziness occurs during exercise, slow down gradually and stop exercising. If you still feel dizzy, lie down with your knees bent. Take your pulse. Check for an irregular heartbeat and/or a fast heart rate. Notify your doctor immediately. If you have not eaten in four hours, you may have low blood sugar. Drink juice or another quick sugar source and eat crackers or drink milk. This prevents a sudden rise followed by a sudden drop in your blood sugar level.

Remember that on some days exercise will be easier than on others. This is normal. One day you will feel great, and the next day the exercise will be more difficult. In addition to experiencing these day-to-day variations in how you feel, other factors such as stress, fatigue, and your emotional state can also affect your response to exercise. On these "off" days, reduce your exercise intensity and duration, or skip your workout for that day. There are also other circumstances when you should plan to reduce or omit exercise.

## When to Reduce or Omit Exercise

Do not exercise when you are sick or injured. This causes too much stress on your body and may lengthen your recovery time. Additionally, do not exercise if you experience any of these symptoms:

- illness and/or fever
- increased chest pain, shortness of breath, or extreme fatigue
- joint or muscle strain, swelling or redness
- severe sunburn
- severe emotional stress
- alcohol hangover

If these symptoms are new or prolonged, consult your doctor for treatment and a recommendation on when to return to exercise.

## EXERCISE GUIDELINES FOR INDIVIDUALS WITH DIABETES

For individuals with diabetes, an exercise program will affect blood sugar levels. This may result in a need to plan medication, meals, and snacks around exercise times. Adjustment in medication doses may be necessary as your exercise program progresses. Following these guidelines will help to keep your blood sugar levels balanced:

1. Check your blood sugar before and after exercise. If your pre-exercise blood sugar is below 100 mg/dl you will need to eat a

snack. If your pre-exercise blood sugar is consistently 300mg/dl or higher, this is a sign that your blood sugar levels are not well controlled. In this case, you should consult your doctor.

2. When you exercise depends on your meal and medication schedule. Try to exercise when your blood sugar is high or slightly above normal, such as one to two hours after a meal. Adjust your diet and/or medication schedule as advised by your doctor. This may involve increasing your carbohydrate intake or decreasing your insulin dose for a specific amount of exercise.

3. Try to exercise at about the same time each day. Avoid exercise during periods of peak insulin activity. This may result in a low blood sugar reaction.

4. Inject insulin in an area (such as the abdomen) that is not active during exercise. Injections to active muscles cause faster absorption by your body and may lower your blood sugar too quickly.

5. Avoid exercise when signs and symptoms of hypoglycemia (blood sugar less than 60mg/dl) or hyperglycemia (blood sugar greater than 300 mg/dl) are present. Mild symptoms of low blood sugar include nervousness, heavy sweating, shakiness and trembling, pale and clammy skin, hunger, blurred or double vision, and rapid heart rate; moderate symptoms include tiredness, short temper, confusion, and personality change; severe symptoms include unconsciousness and coma. Low blood sugar is commonly referred to as an insulin reaction. An insulin reaction may be caused by taking too much insulin (or oral agent), missing or delaying a meal, not eating enough, or exercising more than is usual for you. If your insulin reactions occur more than once or twice a week, you may need to have your meal plan or medication schedule adjusted.

6. Avoid exercising in extreme weather conditions. This can increase the energy demands on your body and lower your blood sugar.

7. Exercise with a partner or have someone available who knows

you have diabetes and knows how to treat a low blood sugar reaction.

8. Carry an emergency sugar supply with you, such as hard candy or cans of apple or orange juice, in case you experience symptoms of low blood sugar.

9. Wear comfortable shoes that fit properly; break in new shoes carefully to avoid blisters and calluses. Wear cotton socks to avoid excessive perspiration. If an injury to your foot does occur, cleanse your wound thoroughly. Visually inspect your feet every day. If any signs of infection (redness, swelling, drainage, pain, or red streak) develop, call your doctor immediately.

10. Wear identification indicating you have diabetes.

11. Avoid exercise when you are ill. Conditions such as a cold, the flu, infection, muscle aches, or a high temperature (above 101 degrees Fahrenheit) can change your insulin requirements and place an added strain on your body.

12. Your blood sugar after exercise should be at least 80mg/dl. If it is not, an additional snack may be needed.

The information presented in this section is a general guideline only. Specific instructions concerning your insulin dose and schedule, your meal quantities and times, and your exercise plan should be discussed in greater detail with your doctor.


## STRENGTH TRAINING

Strength training is a valuable addition to a fitness program because it improves muscle strength and endurance. Combining a strength training program with an aerobic exercise regimen will help you to resume your normal activities, vocation, and recreational pursuits sooner than you think.

The advantages of weight training in terms of your overall health include lower blood pressure, higher HDL or "good cholesterol" levels, stronger bones, better blood sugar control, and improved balance and flexibility.

## Types of Strength Training

There are a variety of strength or resistance training options. Your doctor will recommend the best option for you. The most widely recommended methods for strength training include the following:

- *Body weight:* Lifting your arms or legs (without holding any additional weight) creates enough resistance for a beginner to improve muscle strength. The only resistance here is that of gravity. When this activity loses its challenge for beginners, move to another form of strength training.
- *Elastic rubber bands/tubing:* Based on length, width, and thickness, varying amounts of resistance can be obtained. These elastic bands can be stretched in a variety of directions with the arms and/or legs. In addition to strength gains, this activity will also improve flexibility.
- *Ankle or wrist weights:* These weights wrap around the ankle or wrist (usually with Velcro). An advantage is that the amount of weight can be adjusted based on your ability level. Weights typically range from less than 1 pound to 20 pounds. Start light.
- *Handheld weights:* These are small dumbbell-shaped weights that can be gripped by both hands. They range from 1 to 25 pounds. Handheld weights can be lifted in a variety of directions. The disadvantage of this method is that leg strengthening cannot be achieved with handheld weights.
- *Free weights (barbells):* Free weights include different types of single bars with varying weight. This type of weight training is done primarily with the upper body, and involves higher resistance and skill levels. Special training from a health professional is necessary.
- *Weight-training machines:* These machines provide resistance

through chains, pulleys, elastic tension, or hydraulic cylinders. They allow you to strengthen one muscle group at a time and enable you to lift progressively larger amounts of weights. This form of resistance training also requires proper instruction from a health professional.

## Safety and Strength Training

Your doctor should be consulted before beginning any type of strength training program. Strength training may not be appropriate for individuals with uncontrolled high blood pressure, limited heart pumping ability, irregular heart rhythms, or chest pain. For individuals recovering from heart surgery, a period of six to eight weeks is typically recommended before beginning strength training. After a heart attack, a period of two to eight weeks is typically recommended before beginning a strength training program.

## Be Careful

After clearance is received from your doctor, the following guidelines will ensure that your training is performed safely and efficiently:

1. Perform strength training activities two to three days per week on alternate days.
2. Stop exercise if you experience chest discomfort, dizziness, shortness of breath, chest incision discomfort, or feelings of palpitations.
3. Avoid holding your breath. Always exhale when lifting.
4. Start with the lightest weights on each resistive device and attempt to perform ten to twelve repetitions. If you can lift the weight without difficulty, increase your resistance to a higher weight. You should be able to perform each series of repetitions with no strain and little effort before increasing to a higher weight. Do not increase to a higher weight more often than every one to two weeks.

5. Check your pulse rate at regular intervals. If your heart rate is climbing to the maximum of your target heart rate range, reduce the amount of weight you are using.

6. Maintain a loose, comfortable hand grip on the weights at all times.

7. Slow, controlled movements are desirable. Lift the weights to a count of 2 and lower the weights to a count of 4.

8. The number of times you lift the weights will vary. For achieving strength gains, lifting heavier weights with fewer repetitions is recommended, (for example, eight to ten times). For achieving endurance gains, lifting lighter weights with higher repetitions (twelve to fifteen) is recommended.

9. Exercise large muscle groups before small muscle groups. Include exercises for both the upper and lower body.

10. Rest thirty to ninety seconds between each exercise. Keep moving during this period by walking or performing range of motion activities.

Maintain a record of your strength training session that includes the amount of weight lifted, the number of repetitions, and the types of exercises. Refer to this record log prior to your next training session. Copy the weight-training record in Figure 4.3 to help you track your program. Share this information periodically with your doctor.

Most individuals can benefit from a weight-training program, regardless of age. The goal is not to be a bodybuilder, but to improve muscular tone and conditioning to make day-to-day activities easier. A combination of aerobic exercise and strength training will tone and condition your muscles and improve your overall cardiovascular health. Keep in mind that although strength training yields significant benefits, it should not be used as a substitute for your aerobic exercise program.

Keep track of your weekly weight-training routine by charting your progress below. Record the amount of weight lifted, the number of repetitions (the number of times you lift the weight), and the type of exercise performed. Share this useful information with your doctor on your next visit.

| DATE | WEIGHT LIFTED (LBS.) | REPETITIONS | TYPE OF EXERCISE |
|------|---------------------|-------------|------------------|
| 8/15/97 | 35 lbs. | 12 | 3 arm exercises 3 leg exercises |

FIGURE 4.3    Sample Weight-Training Record

**BOUNCING BACK:**
**YOUR WEIGHT-TRAINING PROGRAM**

- Consult with your doctor about starting a strength training program.
- Select the appropriate strength training modality for you.
- Perform weight training two to three times per week on alternate days.
- Begin with light weights and increase to heavier weights when the weight can be lifted for ten to twelve repetitions without difficulty.
- Always exhale when lifting the weight.
- Do not exceed your target heart rate.
- Stop exercise and call your doctor if you have any chest pain, dizziness, shortness of breath, or irregular heart rate.

## FEELING LIKE YOURSELF AGAIN

Exercising regularly is one of the best gifts you can give yourself. It improves the function of your heart, strengthens your muscles, helps to lower your blood pressure, controls your cholesterol levels, and aids in weight reduction. Following a specific exercise plan can help you to look and feel better within eight to twelve weeks.

Staying motivated will be your challenge. Avoid the pitfalls that allow you to rationalize why you should not exercise. There are several myths circulating about exercise. Do not believe them. Exercise does not make you tired. As you become more physically .

fit, exercise gives you more energy. Exercise does not take too much time. Exercising for a minimum of three days each week for about thirty minutes is all the time you need. Age is also not a limitation to exercise. Being sure that you get enough exercise will assist in maintaining good health and a high quality of life as you get older. Finally, you do not have to be athletic to exercise. Just pick an exercise you enjoy and exercise at a level that brings your heart rate into your target range. (See Figure 4.4.)

There are several ways to stay motivated. Consider exercising with a partner, listening to music, or reading to help keep your interest. Set a scheduled time, note it on your calendar, and consider that time as an appointment you must keep. Add variety to your exercise program by changing your activity periodically. And, finally, reward yourself for meeting your exercise goals. Purchase new equipment or clothes, see a movie, or plan a get-away weekend. Regardless of your age, exercise can become a health habit with benefits that last a lifetime. You will be successful with just a little time management, determination, and creativity.

# WARM-UP EXERCISES

## STANDING EXERCISES FOR UPPER BODY
*(flexibility and strength)*

### ARM CIRCLES

- Stand with feet 12 inches apart. Hold arms out from sides.

- Move arms in forward direction so that arms and hands make 12 inch circles.

- Repeat 10 times. Repeat arm circles in other direction. This time start with one arm pointed up and the other pointed down.

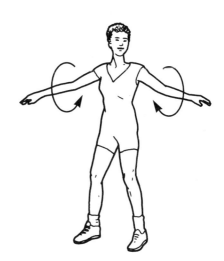

### UPPER BODY TWIST

- Stand tall; feet 18 to 20 inches apart; point feet forward and slightly outward; raise arms out to side (shoulder level).

- Twist upper body to left, keeping arms and hands at shoulder level. Hold 5 seconds and return to starting position. Repeat exercise to the right side.

- Repeat 5 to 8 times.

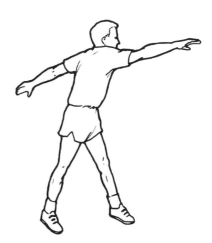

**FIGURE 4.4    Warm-up Exercises and Stretches Your Body Will Love**
Illustrations by Susan Spellman

## WARM-UP EXERCISES

### STANDING EXERCISE FOR TOTAL BODY
*(flexibility and strength)*

#### WINDMILL TOE TOUCHES

- Stand tall; feet apart 18 to 24 inches; arms stretched to sides at shoulder level.

- Bend forward at waist with legs straight. Reach toward right foot with left hand. Reach only as far as you are comfortable (anywhere from your knee to your toe). Return to starting position. Repeat with right hand reaching toward left foot.

- Repeat 10 times.

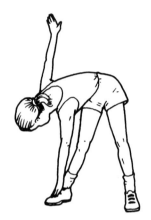

#### LEG LIFTS

- Raise your leg outward away from your body.

- Lower leg.

- Repeat 10 times.

- Change sides.

Hold in each position for 3 to 5 seconds.

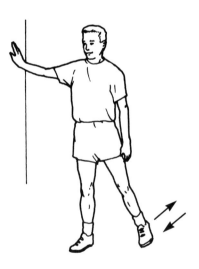

**FIGURE 4.4**    *continued*

# STRETCHES YOUR BODY WILL LOVE

### LEG STRETCH WITH FOOT TO THIGH

- Sit with your left leg in front of you and your right foot to your left thigh.

- Reach down toward the right ankle and hold.

- Sit up straight and relax.

- Repeat.

- Switch leg positions.

- Repeat.

Hold each stretch for 10 to 15 seconds.

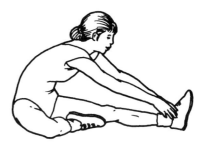

### POINTED TOE STRETCH

- Sit with your legs together.

- Point your toes away from you while reaching toward your ankles (hold).

- Sit up straight and relax.

- Point your toes toward you while reaching toward your ankles (hold).

- Sit up straight and relax.

Hold each stretch for 10 to 15 seconds.

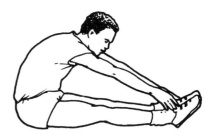

**FIGURE 4.4**    *continued*

## STRETCHES YOUR BODY WILL LOVE

### CALF STRETCH

- Facing a wall, place your right leg straight back and your left leg forward (bend at the knee).

- Press and lean into the wall while keeping your right heel touching the floor.

- Lean in only far enough to feel the calf stretch and hold.

- Switch legs.

- Repeat 4 to 6 times.

Hold each stretch for 10 to 15 seconds.

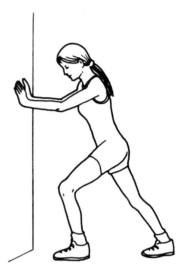

### QUAD STRETCH

- Position yourself facing a wall using one hand for support.

- With your free hand, lift your leg up by your ankle.

Hold each stretch for 10 to 15 seconds.

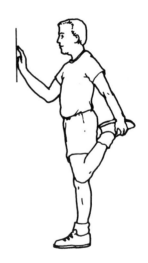

**FIGURE 4.4**    *continued*

## STRETCHES YOUR BODY WILL LOVE

### HIP STRETCH

- Sit with legs straight with floor.

- Cross right foot over left knee and place it on the floor. Hold right knee with left arm and pull it in toward your chest. Turn your head and right shoulder toward the right side and backward. Return to starting position.

- Repeat exercise with left foot crossed over right knee.

- Repeat 1 to 2 times.

Hold each stretch for 10 to 20 seconds.

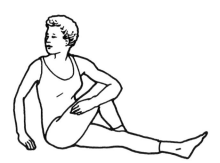

### GROIN STRETCH

- Sit with bottom of feet together. Hold ankles with hands and push knees toward floor with forearms and elbows.

- Pull upper body down toward feet. Return to starting position.

- Repeat 1 to 2 times.

Hold each stretch for 30 seconds.

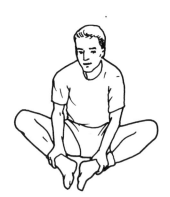

**FIGURE 4.4**    *continued*

## STRETCHES YOUR BODY WILL LOVE

### UPPER BODY STRETCH

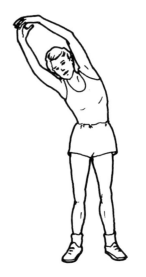

- Reach your arms above your head slowly, lean to your right, and then to your left (repeat 3 to 5 times).

- Be sure to go sideways left and right and not forward or backward.

Hold each stretch for 10 to 15 seconds.

### UPPER BODY SIDE STRETCH

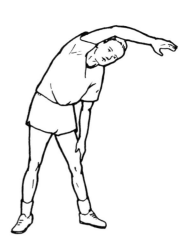

- Stand tall with one arm stretched overhead and other arm down by side; feet 18 to 20 inches apart.

- Bend upper body to the left side as far as you can (not forward or backward, only to side). Return to starting position. Repeat exercise to the right side.

Hold each stretch for 10 to 15 seconds.

**FIGURE 4.4**    *continued*

§

## CHAPTER FIVE

# TAKING CHARGE OF YOUR DIET

THIS IS A TAKE-CHARGE CHAPTER. WHAT YOU EAT AFFECTS MANY risk factors that contribute to heart disease: cholesterol levels, weight, high blood pressure, diabetes, and exercise. Achieving control of your diet will put you in control of your heart disease.

This is not a chapter about diet. It is information about healthy eating. Think about any living object that needs nourishment. When you plant flowers in your garden, you can choose to just water them; they may live but they will never reach their full potential for height or fullness, or produce the buds and flowers you had hoped for. On the other hand, if you research what nutrients and supplements, soil type, and watering schedule they like, they will flourish, producing numerous buds and flowers. They will be strong enough to face any obstacles, such as bad weather or insect infestation. They will probably live beyond their expected life span.

Your diet should include the variety of nutrients needed for you to thrive and become strong enough to face any future obstacles. To begin, you need to review your diet and assess your food preferences and eating patterns. What are the foods you crave? What is lacking in your diet? What times of day do you have the greatest appetite? This review will help you understand your eating behaviors.

You can then focus on how you can meet your appetite demands while sticking to a heart-healthy diet. Chapter 2 provided information on how to determine how many calories and grams of fat you need daily, depending on your trying to lose weight or maintain it. With this knowledge, and committing to the following seven rules, you are on your way to meeting your daily nutritional needs.

1. Total daily calories less than 30 percent from fat.
2. Total daily calories less than 10 percent from saturated fat.
3. Less than 300 mg of cholesterol daily.
4. Less than 3,000 mg of sodium daily.
5. No more than two servings of alcohol daily (2 ounces hard liquor; 7 ounces wine; 17 ounces beer).
6. No more than 200 mg caffeine daily (equivalent to two 8-ounce cups of coffee/day).
7. Six to eight glasses of water daily.

(*Note:* Depending on your medical history, your doctor may recommend other, more specific, diet instructions.)

### NOTE TO FAMILY AND FRIENDS

A heart-healthy diet is not just for individuals with heart disease. Following the guidelines presented in this chapter will help protect you from developing heart disease and other chronic illnesses associated with a poor diet. Making permanent changes for all family members will help to ensure future good health for everyone.

## THE FOOD GUIDE PYRAMID

The food guide pyramid presents the minimum servings of food from each food group that ensures you are consuming a well-balanced diet. Instead of focusing on what you can't have, direct your attention to what you need to eat every day to meet minimum nutritional requirements. (See Figure 5.1.)

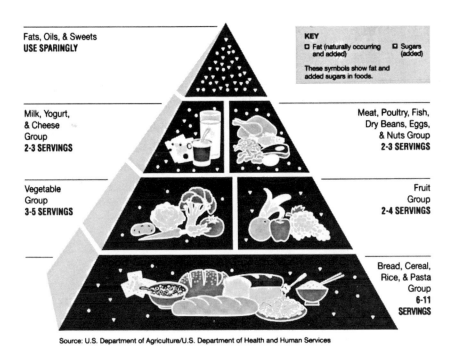

Source: U.S. Department of Agriculture/U.S. Department of Health and Human Services

FIGURE 5.1    Food Guide Pyramid: A Guide to Daily Food Choices

## PROTEIN

The protein serving at the evening meal used to take up more than half of the plate. Now we know we should fill our plates with bread, pasta, rice, vegetables, and fruit. The protein serving should be no more than 3 ounces, or about the size of a deck of playing cards or the palm of a woman's hand. Two 3-ounce servings is all that is needed daily. Protein is essential to build body tissues and produce important enzymes and hormones. The protein we eat cannot be stored by the body, so we need to provide a new supply daily. The simple fact, however, is that we eat much more than our bodies need.

### Animal Products

Animal products are the most common sources of protein but are high in fat, saturated fat, and cholesterol. You don't have to avoid all meat to be healthy. You can reduce the fat content by trimming visible fat; purchasing lean cuts of meat; removing the skin from chicken and turkey; and roasting, grilling, or baking meat on a rack so fat can drip away. Avoid meat in which you can see visible fat, such as sausages (60 to 80 percent of its total calories come from fat) and hotdogs.

### Fish

Fish provides low-fat and usually low-calorie choices for protein. It is recommended that a minimum of two servings of fish be consumed weekly. Shellfish such as shrimp also can be a good source of protein. Although shellfish tends to be high in cholesterol (about 80 mg of cholesterol in 3 ounces), it is low in saturated fat and calories. Eating 3 ounces of shellfish one to two times per week is acceptable.

There have been many reports in the media that consuming fish as a primary source of protein can actually reduce cholesterol. Researchers have found that populations that eat fish as their primary source of protein have a low incidence of coronary heart disease. The theory is that these fish have a high concentration of omega 3 fatty acids, which may reduce cholesterol and interfere with the formation of plaque and blood clots. (See Table 5.1.) Research continues on this topic. However, fish is considered a healthy choice because it is low in fat, low in cholesterol, and low in calories compared to other protein sources. For these reasons, a diet that includes fish at a minimum of two servings per week may result in lower cholesterol levels.

**TABLE 5.1     Sources of Omega 3 Fatty Acids**

|  | GRAMS PER 4 OUNCES |
|---|---|
| Chinook salmon (canned) | 3.3 |
| Chinook salmon (fresh) | 2.4 |
| Atlantic mackerel | 2.5 |
| Pink salmon | 2.2 |
| American eel | 1.9 |
| Coho salmon (canned) | 1.8 |
| Sable fish | 1.7 |
| Tuna | 1.6 |
| Atlantic herring | 1.3 |
| Norwegian sardines | 1.3 |
| Rainbow trout | 1.2 |
| Lake whitefish | 1.0 |
| Pacific oyster | 1.0 |
| **COMPARE WITH:** | |
| Chicken | .03 |
| Lean round steak | Trace |
| Ground beef | Trace |

## Vegetarian Protein Options

Beans (kidney, black, lima, navy, and garbanzo), legumes (peas, lentils, and soybeans), and tofu are good low-fat sources of protein, similar to animal protein. Also, nearly all green, yellow, and starchy vegetables, and flour and cereal products contain some protein. Vegetarian meals using beans, legumes, or tofu also will help to decrease the amount of fat and cholesterol in your diet.

One issue to keep in mind is that not all vegetables, flour, or cereals offer a complete protein source. The body breaks down protein into amino acids that are used as building blocks in the body. The body produces eleven amino acids and obtains the other nine it needs from the diet. Most animal proteins are complete proteins; this means they contain all nine necessary amino acids. Most vegetable proteins are incomplete and must be combined with other protein sources. Table 5.2 gives examples of how to combine protein sources to ensure that you are consuming complete protein.

## Nuts and Seeds

Nuts and seeds are rich sources of vegetable protein, but are high in fat and calories. Limit servings from this group to one serving daily. As noted in Table 5.2, they are a good complement to incomplete protein sources to form a complete protein.

## Food Preparation

How you cook your protein sources also will make a difference in the amount of fat present in your diet. Trim visible fat and skin from meat. Prepare foods by baking, broiling, roasting, or grilling, rather than frying. Be creative with sauces, gravies, and marinades that are low fat. When a recipe requires that you sauté food, use a nonstick pan or fat-free cooking spray. Drain any extra fat after browning meat. Marinating low-fat meats will help to maintain ten-

**TABLE 5.2  Combining Protein Sources to Achieve a Complete Protein**

| | |
|---|---|
| RICE WITH: | 1. Wheat |
| | 2. Legumes |
| | 3. Sesame seeds |
| WHEAT WITH: | 1. Legumes |
| | 2. Soybeans and peanuts |
| | 3. Soybeans and sesame seeds |
| | 4. Rice and soybeans |
| LEGUMES WITH: | 1. Corn |
| | 2. Rice |
| | 3. Wheat |
| | 4. Sesame seeds |
| | 5. Barley |
| | 6. Oats |

derness, in addition to providing a tasty low-fat alternative to heavy sauces and condiments. Remember, low-fat proteins combined with low-fat cooking make for a low-fat body and a healthy heart.

## CARBOHYDRATES

Carbohydrates are the body's primary source of energy, providing fuel to the brain, central nervous system, and muscles. They are listed at the bottom two levels of the food pyramid because they should be the primary source of calories in the diet. Carbohydrates, including grains, fruits, and vegetables, are low in fat and rich in nutrients. Your diet should include six to eleven servings of grains daily (bread, pasta, rice, cereal), two to three servings of fruit, and three to five servings of vegetables daily. Fifty-five percent of your total calories should come from carbohydrates.

## Grains

Grains include breads, cereals, pasta, rice, and legumes. These are naturally low-fat, low-cholesterol, high-fiber foods. Be selective when adding toppings to these foods because this is what usually adds fat and cholesterol.

## Fruits and Vegetables

Fruits and vegetables are low in fat and calories and rich in carbohydrates, vitamins, minerals, and fiber. Most of us do not meet the minimum number of two to three servings of fruits and three to five servings of vegetables daily. At a minimum, fruit should be included at breakfast and lunch, and one serving of vegetables should be eaten at lunch (adding lettuce and tomatoes to your sandwich, or selecting a side salad rather than french fries), and two servings of vegetables at dinner (salad and steamed vegetables). Fruits and vegetables are a good option for snacks, providing a quick energy source without the additional fat calories typically found in chips, cookies, or candy. Fruits and vegetables also have a high water content, providing bulk and a feeling of fullness that helps prevent overeating.

## Fiber

You probably have heard of all the benefits from fiber-rich diets, including lower cholesterol, prevention of constipation, and reduced risk of cancer. What is this miracle food? Fiber is a plant material that cannot be digested. Fiber can be water soluble (oats, fruits, seeds, dried peas, and beans) or water insoluble (nuts, grains, and vegetables). High-fiber foods are low in fat, filling, and add roughage to the body, thus aiding in digestion and elimination (see Table 5.3).

Researchers have found that soluble fiber seems to aid in lowering total blood cholesterol and LDL cholesterol by approximately 3 to 5 percent. Insoluble fiber travels through the digestive tract faster and helps prevent or relieve constipation. The recommended total amount of fiber in the diet daily is 20 to 25 grams. Following the food guide pyramid of two to three servings of fruit, three to five servings of vegetables, and six to eleven servings of carbohydrates will help to insure that you are consuming 20 to 25 grams of fiber daily.

**TABLE 5.3**    **Fiber Content in Foods**

| FOOD | GRAMS OF FIBER |
|---|---|
| **FRUITS** | |
| Blackberries (½ cup) | 4.0 |
| Apple* (1 medium) | 3.5 |
| Pear* (1 medium) | 3.1 |
| Banana (1 medium) | 3.0 |
| Strawberries (1 cup) | 3.0 |
| Blueberries (½ cup) | 3.0 |
| Orange (1) | 2.6 |
| Prunes (2) | 2.0 |
| Peach* (1) | 1.9 |
| **VEGETABLES (⅔ cup)** | |
| Corn | 6.2 |
| Brussels sprouts | 3.5 |
| Carrots | 3.1 |
| Potatoes, cooked | 3.1 |
| Broccoli | 2.9 |
| Spinach | 2.8 |
| Zucchini | 2.4 |

*continued on next page*

**TABLE 5.3** *continued*

| FOOD | GRAMS OF FIBER |
|------|----------------|
| **CEREALS (1 ounce)** | |
| All Bran w/ Extra Fiber | 14 |
| Fiber One + | 13 |
| 100 % Bran | 10 |
| Bran Buds | 10 |
| Shredded Wheat (2 biscuits) | 6.1 |
| Grape-Nuts | 5.0 |
| Oats, rolled (½ cup) | 4.5 |
| **BREADS** | |
| Bran muffin (1) | 4.0 |
| Whole-wheat bread (2 slices) | 3.2 |
| Pumpernickel bread (2 slices) | 3.2 |
| Rye bread ( 2 slices) | 2.8 |
| Cracked-wheat bread (2 slices) | 2.4 |
| **GRAINS** | |
| Rice, brown (⅔ cup) | 3.0 |
| Barley, dry (⅔ cup) | 2.1 |
| Rice, white (⅔ cup) | 1.1 |
| **LEGUMES** | |
| Lentils, cooked (½ cup) | 9.0 |
| Kidney beans, cooked (½ cup) | 9.7 |
| Pinto beans, cooked (½ cup) | 8.9 |
| Lima beans, cooked (½ cup) | 7.4 |

* With skin.

Source: United States Department of Agriculture (USDA)

## DAIRY PRODUCTS

Consumer demand for low-fat dairy products has been met. Dairy products no longer have to be a significant source of fat in your diet. Choosing skim milk and low-fat or fat-free cheeses and yogurt will help you to get the nutritional benefits without the added fat.

Dairy products are a significant source of calcium and protein. There are other sources of calcium besides dairy products. These include broccoli, dark green leafy vegetables, tofu, beans, peas, lentils, and canned fish with soft edible bones.

Most of us know that calcium is important for building and maintaining bones and teeth. Calcium also has other functions in the body, including helping to regulate the heartbeat, helping muscles grow and contract, helping the blood to clot, and helping the body to use iron. The recommended servings from the dairy group is 1,000 mg daily, which should be increased for pregnant and lactating women and teenagers to 1,200 to 1,500 mg daily. (See Table 5.4.)

TABLE 5.4    Dairy Comparison

| 8-OZ. SERVING SIZE | TOTAL CALORIES | % OF CALORIES FROM FAT | MILLIGRAMS OF CALCIUM |
|---|---|---|---|
| Whole milk | 150 | 51 | 288 |
| 2% milk | 125 | 38 | 287 |
| 1% milk | 104 | 22 | 300 |
| Skim milk | 81 | 2 | 302 |

## FATS, OILS, AND SWEETS

At the top of the food pyramid are the fats, oils, and sweets. These should be eaten in limited quantities because they are high in calories (one fat gram equals 9 calories, whereas one carbohydrate gram equals 4 calories), and can be high in saturated fat, which raises cholesterol.

There are three types of fat: saturated, polyunsaturated, and monounsaturated. Saturated fats such as fatty cuts of meat, whole-milk dairy products, butter, palm oil, and coconut oil, raise cholesterol levels and increase the risk of blockages developing along vessel lining walls. Polyunsaturated fats such as corn and safflower oils, and monounsaturated fats such as olive and peanut oils, are a better choice for cooking because they do not raise cholesterol levels and may even raise the HDL ("good") cholesterol. However, even these should be used sparingly.

Your body does have use for dietary fat. You need about 1 to 2 percent polyunsaturated fat (usually in the form of vegetable oil) daily as a source of the essential fatty acid called linoleic acid and also to transport certain fat-soluble vitamins through the walls of the digestive tract. Without fat you would not absorb vitamins A, D, E, and K. You are able to meet these needs with just 1 tablespoon of polyunsaturated fat, but the average American adult consumes about 6 to 8 tablespoons of fat daily. In general, no more than 10 percent of your total calories should come from saturated fat, and no more than 20 to 30 percent of your total calories should come from fat.

Americans are snacking more than ever. It is estimated that about half our total calorie intake is snack or convenience foods. So how do we control these snack attacks? You can first try to prevent the cravings from occurring. This can be done by eating high-fiber foods that are low in fat and calories and give you a feeling of fullness. Drinking six to eight glasses of water daily will also help to control snacking impulses. Choosing low-fat snack options will help to control calorie and fat intake. Consider fruits, fresh vegetables, low-fat popcorn, pretzels, rice cakes, gelatin, fruit sorbet, low-fat yogurt, whole-grain cereals, breads, and bagels as choices. Finally, if these substitutes won't do, consider eating half a serving of the desired food by sharing with a friend or asking for a smaller portion size. Remember, moderation is the key to success, but planning your indulgences will help you stay in control. Totally depriving yourself of a food you enjoy may result in overeating.

## EXPLORING THE WORLD OF HEALTHY EATING

### Food Labels

Following a low fat diet begins with increasing your awareness of serving size and the fat, cholesterol, and calorie content of foods. In 1993, the Food and Drug Administration made this easier by introducing new food labels called "Nutrition Facts" on food products. This information provides serving size, calories, total carbohydrates, dietary fiber, protein, vitamins and minerals, total fat, saturated fat, cholesterol, and sodium, and presents recommended daily values based on a 2,000 and 2,500 calorie per day diet.

Review chapter 2 to determine your daily calorie and fat budget. With this in mind, reviewing food labels will help you to stay within your allotted limits based on serving size, calorie total, and fat content. The new labels are designed to help you make informed choices about food. (See Figure 5.2.)

Understanding other claims advertised on food packaging will also help you make knowledgeable decisions. (See Table 5.5.)

Even with the new federally mandated food labeling, there is potential to be misled by advertisers. A company may advertise, for example, that a product is cholesterol free. Although it may be

## SERVING SIZE

Is your serving the same size as the one on the label? If you eat double the serving size listed, you need to double the nutrient and calorie values. If you eat one-half the serving size shown here, cut the nutrient and calorie values in half.

## CALORIES

Are you overweight? Cut back a little on calories! Look here to see how a serving of the food adds to your daily total. A 5'4", 138-lb. active woman needs about 2,200 calories each day. A 5'10", 174-lb. active man needs about 2,900. How about you?

## TOTAL CARBOHYDRATE

When you cut down on fat, you can eat more carbohydrates. Carbohydrates are in foods like bread, potatoes, fruits, and vegetables. Choose these often! They give you nutrients and energy.

## DIETARY FIBER

Grandmother called it "roughage," but her advice to eat more is still up-to-date! That goes for both soluble and insoluble kinds of dietary fiber. Fruits, vegetables, whole-grain foods, beans, and peas are all good sources and can help reduce the risk of heart disease and cancer.

## PROTEIN

Most Americans get more protein than they need. Where there is animal protein, there is also fat and cholesterol. Eat small servings of lean meat, fish, and poultry. Use skim or low-fat milk, yogurt, and cheese. Try vegetable proteins like beans, grains, and cereals.

## VITAMINS AND MINERALS

Your goal here is 100% if each for the day. Don't count on one food to do it all. Let a combination of foods add up to a winning score.

# Nutrition Facts

Serving Size ½ cup (114g)
Servings Per Container 4

## Amount Per Serving

| Calories 90 | Calories from Fat 30 |
|---|---|
| | **% Daily Value*** |
| **Total Fat** 3g | 5% |
| Saturated Fat 0g | 0% |
| **Cholesterol** 0mg | 0% |
| **Sodium** 300mg | 13% |
| **Total Carbohydrate** 13g | 4% |
| Dietary Fiber 3g | 12% |
| Sugars 3g | |
| **Protein** 3g | |

| | | | |
|---|---|---|---|
| Vitamin A | 80% | • Vitamin C | 60% |
| Calcium | 4% | • Iron | 4% |

* Percent Daily Values are based on a 2,000 calorie diet. Your daily values may be higher or lower depending on your calorie needs:

| | Calories | 2,000 | 2,500 |
|---|---|---|---|
| Total Fat | Less than | 65g | 80g |
| Sat Fat | Less than | 20g | 25g |
| Cholesterol | Less than | 300mg | 300mg |
| Sodium | Less than | 2,400mg | 2,400mg |
| Total Carbohydrate | | 300g | 375g |
| Fiber | | 25g | 30g |

Calories per gram:
Fat 9 • Carbohydrate 4 • Protein 4

More nutrients may be listed on some labels.

## TOTAL FAT

Aim low: Most people need to cut back on fat! Too much fat may contribute to heart disease and cancer. Try to limit your **calories from fat**. For a healthy heart, choose foods with a big difference between the total number of calories and the number of calories from fat.

## SATURATED FAT

A new kind of fat? No—saturated fat is part of the total fat in food. It is listed separately because it's the key player in raising blood cholesterol and your risk of heart disease. Eat less!

## CHOLESTEROL

Too much cholesterol—a second cousin to fat—can lead to heart disease. Challenge yourself to eat less than 300 mg each day.

## SODIUM

You call it "salt," the label calls it "sodium." Either way, it may add up to high blood pressure in some people. So, keep your sodium intake low—2,400 to 3,000 mg or less each day.*

## DAILY VALUE

Feel like you're drowning in numbers? Let the Daily Value be your guide. Daily Values are listed for people who eat 2,000 or 2,500 calories each day. If you eat more, your personal daily value may be higher than what's listed on the label. If you eat less, your personal daily value may be lower.

For fat, saturated fat, cholesterol and sodium, choose foods with a low **% Daily Value**. For total carbohydrate, dietary fiber, vitamins and minerals, your daily value goal is to reach 100% of each.

g=grams (About 28 g=1 ounce)
mg=miligrams (1,000 mg=1 g)

*The AHA recommends no more than 3,000 mg sodium per day for healthy adults.*

cholesterol free, it might still contain saturated fat. As we have discussed, saturated fat should be viewed with alarm because of its effect on increasing cholesterol levels. Foods identified as fat free may have higher sugar and calorie contents than conventional products to compensate for the loss of flavor due to the absence of fat. This is a concern if you are trying to lose weight, or have diabetes and/or elevated triglyceride levels.

**TABLE 5.5    Interpreting Food Labels**

| | |
|---|---|
| **FAT FREE** | Less than 0.5 grams of fat per serving |
| **LOW FAT** | 3 grams of fat (or less) per serving |
| **LEAN** | Less than 10 grams of fat, 4.5 grams of saturated fat, and no more than 95 mg of cholesterol per serving |
| **EXTRA LEAN** | Less than 5 grams of fat, 2 grams of saturated fat, and 95 mg of cholesterol per serving |
| **LIGHT** | ⅓ less calories or no more than ½ the fat of the higher-calorie, higher-fat version; or no more than ½ the sodium of the higher-sodium version |
| **CHOLESTEROL FREE** | Less than 2 mg of cholesterol and 2 grams (or less) of saturated fat per serving |
| **REDUCED SODIUM** | At least 25% less sodium per serving |

## FOOD PREPARATION

The method you use to prepare your food will make a difference in the number of calories and percent of fat in the meal. A heart-healthy diet does not mean you have to give up your favorite recipes. Following the simple menu substitutions in Table 5.6 shows how to modify traditional favorite recipes to improve their nutritional benefits.

TABLE 5.6    Menu Substitutions

| WHEN A RECIPE CALLS FOR: | SUBSTITUTE: |
| --- | --- |
| Solid shortening or lard | Liquid vegetable oil or margarine |
| Oil | Bananas or applesauce (equal amounts) |
| Sour Cream | Fat-free plain yogurt |
| | Low-fat cottage cheese blended until smooth |
| | Ricotta cheese made from skim milk |
| | Chilled evaporated skim milk with 1 tsp. lemon juice |
| Whole Milk | Skim milk (1 cup whole = 1 cup skim) |
| | Nonfat dry milk |
| Chocolate | 1 tbsp. cocoa + 3 tbsp. polyunsaturated oil |
| Eggs | Substitute cholesterol-free egg substitute |
| | ¼ cup for one large egg |
| | Substitute 2 egg whites for 1 whole egg |
| Cream Cheese | Fat-free cream cheese |
| Fudge Sauce | Chocolate sauce (0% fat) |
| Sugars | Reduce by one-third to one-half |
| Salt | Reduce by one-half or eliminate |

## Savor the Flavor: Using Spices to Flavor Food

Cooking with seasonings rather than salt can help to control your sodium intake and flavor your food without adding extra fat or calories. Table 5.7 will guide you in enhancing your recipes.

**TABLE 5.7    Seasoning Substitutions**

**ALLSPICE**  Lean ground meats, stews, tomatoes, peaches, apple-sauce, cranberry sauce, gravies, lean meat

**ALMOND EXTRACT**  Puddings, fruits

**BASIL**  Fish, lamb, lean ground meats, stews, salads, soups, sauces, fish cocktails

**BAY LEAVES**  Lean meats, stews, poultry, soups, tomatoes

**CARAWAY SEEDS**  Lean meats, stews, soups, salads, breads, cabbage, asparagus, noodles

**CHIVES**  Salads, sauces, soups, lean meats, vegetables

**CIDER VINEGAR**  Salads, vegetables, sauces

**CINNAMON**  Fruits ( especially apples), breads, pie crusts

**CURRY POWDER**  Lean meats (especially lamb), veal, chicken, fish, tomatoes, tomato soup, mayonnaise

**DILL**  Fish sauces, soups, tomatoes, cabbages, carrots, cauliflower, green beans, cucumbers, potatoes, salads, macaroni, lean beef, lamb, chicken, fish

**GARLIC** (not garlic salt)  Lean meats, fish, soups, salads, vegetables, tomatoes, potatoes

**GINGER**  Chicken, fruits

**LEMON JUICE**  Lean meats, fish, poultry, salads, vegetables

**MACE**  Hot breads, apples, fruits, salads, carrots, cauliflower, squash, potatoes, veal, lamb

**MUSTARD (dry)**  Lean ground meats, lean meats, chicken, fish, salads, asparagus, broccoli, Brussels sprouts, cabbage, mayonnaise, sauces

**NUTMEG**  Fruits, pie crust, lemonade, potatoes, chicken, fish, lean meat loaf, toast, veal, pudding

**ONION** (not onion salt)  Lean meats, stews, vegetables, salads, soups

*continued on next page*

**TABLE 5.7** *continued*

---

**PAPRIKA** Lean meats, fish, soups, salads, sauces, vegetables

**PARSLEY** Lean meats, fish, soups, salads, sauces, vegetables

**PEPPERMINT EXTRACT** Fruits, puddings

**PIMIENTO** Salads, vegetables, casserole dishes

**ROSEMARY** Chicken, veal, lean meat loaf, lean beef, lean pork, sauces, stuffing, potatoes, peas, lima beans

**SAGE** Lean meats, stews, biscuits, tomatoes, green beans, fish, lima beans, onions, lean pork

**SAVORY** Salads, lean pork, lean ground meats, soups, green beans, squash, tomatoes, lima beans, peas

**TURMERIC** Lean meats, fish, sauces, rice

**THYME** Lean meats ( especially veal and pork), sauces, soups, onions, peas, tomatoes, salads

---

## Stocking Your Kitchen

A well-stocked kitchen will help you to stick with your low-fat eating plan. Take inventory of what you have available. Foods listed in Table 5.8 should be available in your refrigerator, freezer, and pantry shelves.

## YOUR GUIDE TO EATING OUT

At home we have control of what we eat, how much we eat, and how it is prepared. This is the ideal. However, many of us live in two-career or single-parent families with lengthy work hours, long commutes, and little time to plan, shop for, and prepare meals. This is why the restaurant business is thriving.

**TABLE 5.8    Stocking Your Kitchen**

**PROTEIN**

Lean meat choices:    Poultry—skinless turkey, chicken
Beef—round tip, top round, eye of round,
top loin, tenderloin, sirloin
Pork—tenderloin, boneless lean ham,
center loin chop
Fish—limit shellfish to one serving per week

Beans, legumes
Eggs (egg substitute or 2 egg whites = 1 egg)

**FRUITS AND VEGETABLES**

Variety of fresh fruits and vegetables
Canned low-sodium fruits, vegetables
Frozen vegetables
Canned tomatoes and tomato paste

**CARBOHYDRATES**

Whole-grain bread
Pasta and noodles
Ready-to-eat cereals
Rice
Popcorn, pretzels

**DAIRY PRODUCTS**

Skim milk
Low-fat or fat-free yogurt, cottage cheese
Nonfat frozen yogurt

**FATS, OILS, AND CONDIMENTS**

Low-fat or fat-free salad dressings and mayonnaise
Low-fat margarine
Vinegar
Spices
Olive oil and/or vegetable oil
Mustard, ketchup

A closer look at your schedule may help you understand what your eating patterns are. You may find that better planning will help you to eat more meals at home. However, when you do find it necessary to eat out, this doesn't mean you have to eat high-fat, high-sodium, high-calorie meals. More restaurants are responding to consumer demand to hold the fat while maintaining the taste. Armed with a little knowledge, you can make heart-healthy choices.

*Fast food:* Select grilled chicken or a small hamburger or roast beef sandwich. Use lettuce, tomato, onion, ketchup, and/or mustard as condiments. Have a side salad with fat-free salad dressing or a plain baked potato. Avoid burgers topped with cheese, mayonnaise-based dressings, bacon, and french fries. (A Burger King Whopper with cheese has 45 grams of fat!)

*Steakhouses:* Select a 3- to 6-ounce steak (choose low-fat protein for other meals the rest of the day). Lean cuts of steak include London broil, filet mignon, round or flank steak, sirloin tip, and tenderloin. Accompany meals with a baked potato or rice and salad with low-fat or fat-free dressing on the side. Avoid fatty cuts of meat such as rib eye, porterhouse, and T-bone steaks; Caesar salad; and fried vegetables.

*Italian:* Pasta is inherently low fat. The key to keeping your meal heart healthy is to select low-fat sauces such as marsala or marinara sauce. Avoid cheese- and meat-filled pasta and cream sauces.

*Mexican:* Select grilled chicken (chicken fajitas) or fish. Skip the tortilla chips, sour cream, and guacamole.

*Chinese:* Choose stir-fried or steamed dishes with chicken, fish, and vegetables. Avoid deep-fried items such as egg rolls.

*French:* Select entrées that use wine and olive oil rather than butter and cream. A good choice is poached or broiled fish. Skip the rich desserts or share one with a friend.

In general, choose items that are poached, steamed, broiled, and roasted. Ask your waiter to serve sauces and salad dressings on the side. Make one selection from the bread basket. Avoid fatty condiments such as sour cream. For dessert, select fresh fruit, or opt to share a dessert with other guests. Low-fat eating does not mean you have to give up tasty foods—you just need to be selective. Bon appetit!

## TAKING CONTROL

You are in control. Are you giving your body everything it needs to operate efficiently? Just as you feed the flowers in your garden, are you feeding yourself everything you need to achieve optimum physical and emotional health?

Treating your body to a healthy, well-balanced diet will decrease your risk for future heart problems by helping to control weight, cholesterol, and blood sugar levels. There are times when the hustle and bustle of daily living requires that you prepare quick, convenient meals. You now know how to do this in a wholesome way. Understanding what the healthiest options are in a variety of eating situations will help you be prepared, whether you are stopping for lunch at a fast-food restaurant or at a business meeting at the local steakhouse. You know how to select a healthy meal from a variety of menus.

A balanced diet will do more than help you to increase your overall health. Your skin tone will improve, your hair will be healthier, and you may even notice your disposition is better. Ask yourself at the end of each day, "Did I take good care of myself today?"

§

## CHAPTER SIX

# KICKING YOUR STRESS HABIT

THIS IS A STORY ABOUT JEAN. SHE IS A FIFTY-FOUR-YEAR-OLD WOMAN who had a heart attack and three PTCAs in one year. Jean is not where she thought she would be at this age. Prior to the onset of health problems she was married, worked long hours for many years at a job she liked, and spent time with family and friends. Life was good (stress free she thought) until she woke up one morning with chest pain. Thinking it was heartburn, she took a shower and got dressed. At this point, in addition to the pain, she was sweating and experiencing numbness. Jean went to the hospital and was told she was having a heart attack. Three days later, she underwent her first PTCA with atherectomy. The following day, she underwent a second PTCA with stent placement. The next three months were spent recovering. Undaunted, Jean returned to work and took up her life where she left off.

Things were going smoothly until her husband died suddenly of an asthma attack. Jean found herself planning his funeral, settling his business affairs, and facing the prospect of living alone after thirty-five years of companionship. In addition to this, Jean was working for a new boss and was having difficulty juggling her job schedule and getting along with her supervisor. In response to this stress, Jean began to have severe angina attacks. She was diagnosed with another blocked artery and underwent her third PTCA procedure.

Looking back, Jean could see how her stress was building up and affecting her health. She was a recent widow, putting in long hours at an office where morale was low, and taking little time for herself. Jean decided to face her stressors and slow down. She entered a cardiac rehabilitation program, practiced patience (with herself and others), arranged to work at home when she could, focused on her gardening, asked friends and family for help, took a walk to cool down when her temper flared, and made her physical and mental health her first priority. It took concessions and compromises, but Jean is a happier and healthier person for making changes in her life.

## THE CHALLENGE OF STRESS

Stress is a part of life. None of us can keep it from happening, but we can manage how it affects our health. As you may recall from chapter 2, during a stress response, the heart beats faster, blood pressure rises, breathing quickens, perspiration increases, muscles tense, digestion slows, fats and sugars more readily enter the bloodstream, and chemicals are released into the body to make the blood clot easily. Fortunately, our bodies are well equipped to handle a reasonable amount of stress (even with heart disease). Think of this stress response as a normal part of your everyday life. It can be positive (eustress) when it gives you the energy you need to thrive during times of anticipation and excitement, or it can be negative (distress), adversely affecting your health, when it becomes prolonged and unrelenting.

This chapter will guide you in understanding the formula for successful stress management. We will discuss, step by step, how to recognize the warning signs of stress, how to identify coping methods that you may already use, how to adopt additional coping strategies, and how to develop your own stress management plan. You will gain control as you become aware of prolonged stress buildups, as you recognize what you can change to calm yourself quickly, and as you practice your favorite coping strategies on a regular basis.

Stress management involves making lifestyle changes that will help you to reduce the behavioral, physical, mental, and emotional responses commonly associated with stress. The lifestyle changes you make need not be drastic, just sensible. Just as there are many sources of stress, there, too, are many tactics for coping. Coping techniques, how you think and what you do to manage your stress, will help you to restore your equilibrium and sense of control. The methods you will learn involve restructuring your thoughts and practicing relaxation techniques. Your goal is to use these techniques regularly to reduce your stressors before they have time to become cumulative and prolonged. Regular practice will put you in better control of your stress and your health.

## STEP 1:
## RECOGNIZING THE WARNING SIGNS OF STRESS

Becoming aware of how you react to your stressors is the first step toward effective coping. The "Stress Symptom Checklist" in Figure 6.1 lists common difficulties people report while under stress. For each item, place a check in the column that best describes how you have felt or what you have done during the past two months. This checklist is not intended to measure the amount of stress you have in your life; rather, it is a tool for you to use to become conscious of how you tend to react to stressors.

# STRESS SYMPTOM CHECKLIST

**NEV** = Never experienced
**OCC** = Occasionally (once or twice in the past two months)
**OFT** = Often (once or twice every two to three weeks)
**FRE** = Frequently (once or twice a week)
**CON** = Constant occurrence (two or more times per week)

|  | NEV | OCC | OFT | FRE | CON |
|---|---|---|---|---|---|
| **BEHAVIORAL SYMPTOMS:** | | | | | |
| • Sleep difficulties | ___ | ___ | ___ | ___ | ___ |
| • Compulsive eating | ___ | ___ | ___ | ___ | ___ |
| • Loss of appetite | ___ | ___ | ___ | ___ | ___ |
| • Eating poorly | ___ | ___ | ___ | ___ | ___ |
| • Excess smoking | ___ | ___ | ___ | ___ | ___ |
| • Overuse of alcohol | ___ | ___ | ___ | ___ | ___ |
| • Inability to get things done | ___ | ___ | ___ | ___ | ___ |
| • Nervous habits (for example, biting fingernails) | ___ | ___ | ___ | ___ | ___ |
| • Not going to, or late to work | ___ | ___ | ___ | ___ | ___ |
| • Loss of sexual interest | ___ | ___ | ___ | ___ | ___ |
| • Complaining about minor problems | ___ | ___ | ___ | ___ | ___ |
| **PHYSICAL SYMPTOMS\*:** | | | | | |
| • Headaches | ___ | ___ | ___ | ___ | ___ |
| • Stiff or sore neck, shoulders, or low back | ___ | ___ | ___ | ___ | ___ |
| • Heart pounding or racing for no apparent reason | ___ | ___ | ___ | ___ | ___ |

*Remaining after your doctor has ruled out the possibility that these symptoms are related to a physical cause.

**FIGURE 6.1**    **Stress Symptom Checklist**

|  | NEV | OCC | OFT | FRE | CON |
|---|---|---|---|---|---|

## PHYSICAL SYMPTOMS*
*continued:*

- Feelings of nausea,
  indigestion, butterflies
- Sweaty or clammy hands
- Muscle tension
  (neck and shoulders)
- Indigestion, constipation,
  or diarrhea
- Rapid, shallow breathing
  or shortness of breath
- Restlessness or tiring easily

## MENTAL SYMPTOMS:

- Constant worry
- Trouble thinking clearly
- Forgetfulness
- Negative thoughts
  about self
- Difficulty in making
  decisions
- Lack of creativity

## EMOTIONAL SYMPTOMS:

- Feelings of nervousness
  or tension
- Feelings of depression
- Overly sensitive or defensive
- Feelings of guilt or despair
- Irritable and/or easily
  angered

*continued on next page*

**FIGURE 6.1**     *continued*

|  | NEV | OCC | OFT | FRE | CON |
|---|---|---|---|---|---|
| **EMOTIONAL SYMPTOMS** *continued:* | | | | | |
| • Very little laughter or joy | ____ | ____ | ____ | ____ | ____ |
| • Crying or on the verge of tears | ____ | ____ | ____ | ____ | ____ |
| • Feelings of frustration | ____ | ____ | ____ | ____ | ____ |
| • Feelings of helplessness or hopelessness | ____ | ____ | ____ | ____ | ____ |

*Source: David Hyde, Ph.D., Department of Health Education, The University of Maryland, College Park. Adapted and reprinted with permission.*

**FIGURE 6.1**    *continued*

In today's society, with the many responsibilities you face daily, it is likely that you will experience at least some of the stress symptoms in this checklist. However, experiencing multiple symptoms, or one or two on an ongoing basis, could suggest that you are under too much stress and would benefit from taking actions to reduce these stressors in order to prevent future health problems. The starting point of your successful stress management program is identifying your stressors and becoming conscious of how you tend to react to them.

**KICKING YOUR STRESS HABIT**

*Congratulations!* You've completed the first step in better managing your stress:

Step 1 = *recognizing the warning signs of stress*

# STEP 2:
# IDENTIFYING YOUR OWN COPING STRATEGIES

Identifying your own strategies is the second step to effective coping. Chances are you already are practicing several effective coping strategies. Do you know what techniques you practice? What do you do to help yourself relax? List as many strategies as you can think of in Figure 6.2.

WHAT COPING TECHNIQUES DO YOU PRACTICE?

1. _____

2. _____

3. _____

4. _____

5. _____

6. _____

7. _____

8. _____

9. _____

10. _____

**FIGURE 6.2    Coping Strategies Worksheet**

Next, give some additional thought to the two questions in Figure 6.3. Then write your responses in the spaces provided. List at least five experiences or life events that you can recall.

---

**WHAT ARE YOU DOING WHEN YOU FEEL YOUR BEST?**

1. _____
2. _____
3. _____
4. _____
5. _____


**WHAT EXPERIENCES HAVE MADE YOU FEEL POSITIVE ABOUT YOURSELF?**

1. _____
2. _____
3. _____
4. _____
5. _____

---

**FIGURE 6.3**　　**Coping Strategies Worksheet**

If you left any spaces blank, you may need to probe a little more. The following exercise can help you to identify effective coping strategies that you may use automatically, or at least without much thought. Using the chart in Figure 6.4, pick a different four-hour block of time every day of the week to write down what you are doing when you feel your best. Vary the time of day you choose for this exercise (morning, afternoon, evening) in order to obtain a sampling of your routine.

| DAY | TIME | WHAT ARE YOU DOING WHEN YOU FEEL YOUR BEST? WHAT EXPERIENCES MAKE YOU FEEL POSITIVE ABOUT YOURSELF? |
|---|---|---|
| Monday | | |
| Tuesday | | |
| Wednesday | | |
| Thursday | | |
| Friday | | |
| Saturday | | |
| Sunday | | |

FIGURE 6.4    Daily Coping Strategies Worksheet

One of the best ways to manage your stress is to build more of these pleasurable experiences into your life. Repeating your positive experiences and happiest moments, at regular intervals, will help you to stay cool, calm, and in control. Being able to identify these positive strategies will help you to both strengthen and duplicate them.

**KICKING YOUR STRESS HABIT**

*Congratulations!* You have completed the second step in better managing your stress:

Step 2 = *identifying your own coping strategies*

## STEP 3:
## MORE RELIEF IS ON THE WAY!

Your next challenge is to learn new coping strategies that may work when others you have tried have failed. This will improve your coping power! You will find that the more methods you are able to adopt, the greater your reserve of options will be during a period of heightened stress. The best coping tactics are the ones that make you feel relaxed and vibrant. We will begin this section by reviewing some of the best techniques for eliciting a relaxation response: changing your point of view, laughing regularly, managing your environment, working out stress in healthy ways, finding support, finding a spiritual center, and putting things in perspective.

You may find that some of these methods work well for you, and others do not. Try all of them, but adopt only those strategies that are particularly effective for you. Give each some time, however. It takes practice to become skillful. Your approach to managing your stress should be to take the information in this chapter and put a little time and effort aside each day to practice what you have learned. The rewards will follow!

## Change Your Point of View— It's Mind over Matter

How you interpret life events can either make a stress response go away or encourage it to stay indefinitely. The good news is that you get to make this choice. You can choose to counter negative thoughts with positive ones or you can choose to become burdened by the consequences of excess stress and wallow in negative energy. Your thoughts can be your best friend or your worst enemy when it comes to prompting stress. Self-defeating thoughts should be avoided, as they can adversely affect your moods, behaviors, and health.

This section will help you to become conscious of your thought patterns and lays the groundwork for helping you to avoid self-defeating thoughts. Rethinking how you might better respond and reacting differently to a situation or event is the key to stress management. Changing your thoughts takes some practice, so don't get discouraged! Taming an active mind to focus automatically is an acquired skill. Hang on, you'll get there!

A good starting point for learning to focus your mind is to practice a stress management technique called meditation. Meditation is a method of "concentration" that allows you to clear your mind when it becomes cluttered with a lot of information. It's a way of filtering your thoughts—controlling what is coming in and what should go out.

There are many different ways to meditate. One way is to focus on words or phrases as you calmly breathe. For example, "calm down," "things will work out," and "relax." Other ways include performing repetitive physical behaviors (such as slow breathing exercises), listening to repetitive sounds (such as to the sea), holding an object (such as a seashell), or by visually focusing on an image or object (watching the ocean waves). All of these meditation techniques can promote a relaxation response (lowered heart rate, lowered blood pressure, slowed breathing rate, lowered metabolism, and less muscle tension) when performed in a comfortable position in a quiet atmosphere.

In addition to these physical benefits, meditation can clear your mind so that you can become more aware of how your perceptions and behaviors are affecting how you respond to stressful situations. Next time you feel yourself experiencing information overload, use meditation to empty your mind and to focus.

Let's take a look at your ability to focus as you identify your typical reactions to stress in Figure 6.5. For this exercise, we will give you an example stressor. In the spaces provided, write down how you would react physically and mentally to each stressor listed.

Now that you have outlined each response, we will describe how you can change negative thoughts so that your physical and mental reactions to these stressors could be different.

Changing your thought patterns involves getting rid of old, ineffective ways of responding to your stressors and adopting new thought patterns that allow you to better manage your stress and, ultimately, your health. There are four steps to this process:

1. *Awareness*: identifying your stressors and determining your emotional attitude about each one.
2. *Reevaluation*: keeping an open mind about how you might look at your thoughts differently and come up with an alternative way of responding to your stressors.
3. *Adopting a new frame of mind*: turning a new thought into reality by practicing the new thought in place of the old.
4. *Evaluating your new frame of mind*: looking at how successful the new plan is.

If you find that your new way of thinking was not successful for you, try adopting another and another and another until you find the one that works. Here's an example: Let's say you have negative thoughts about your recovery from heart disease. One way of thinking differently may be to change those negative thoughts to positive

## IDENTIFYING YOUR IMMEDIATE THOUGHTS

| EXAMPLE STRESSOR | HOW WOULD YOU REACT MENTALLY AND PHYSICALLY TO THIS STRESSOR? |
|---|---|
| You get cut off on the highway by another driver. | |
| You are at a restaurant, ready to leave, and it seems like you are waiting forever for the check. | |
| You need money at 8 P.M. and your card does not work at the ATM machine. | |
| You are walking to work from the train which was late, horns are blowing, construction crews are jackhammering, and a person running to catch the "walk" signal strongly bumps your shoulder as he goes by. He doesn't say "excuse me." | |
| Your friend or spouse is in the hospital. | |

FIGURE 6.5    Identifying Your Immediate Thoughts

ones. For example, your initial opinion about adopting a new low-fat diet plan may be negative. You may view this lifestyle change as one that will take all the pleasure out of eating. Alternatively, you can restructure this thought by telling yourself that you can continue to eat a variety of the foods you like; you just need to balance your intake of various foods. So, you can eat a hamburger, just not too often! That's perhaps inconvenient, but not catastrophic.

Now that you have learned the steps involved in restructuring your thoughts, let's reexamine the example stressors. Look at Figure 6.6. This time, follow the four-step process for changing your thoughts. Try to adopt a new way of thinking about each stressor.

These changes require time and effort on your part to understand the ways that you normally respond to stress and to make adjustments in your thinking patterns that will lead to effective stress management. Each success will help you realize that many of your old ways of thinking were overreactions. Restructuring your thoughts will help you to see your stressors in a new light. What a difference it makes!

You can also learn to tune into your thoughts by asking yourself these questions: 1) Does your stress typically relate to people, places, events, things, or issues? 2) How do you typically respond to these stressors? 3) Can you think of ways that will help you to respond differently? As you answer these questions, you may discover that you were not previously aware of who, what, when, why, and how your stress is engaged. As you learn to become consciously aware of your thought processes and how you respond to situations, events, and people, you may also find that changing your perspective and your responses may be easier than you think.

As you improve your ability to understand how you think and respond to various situations, your next step will be to learn to react in a positive way. What you tell yourself can actually influence how you respond. Your mind is a powerful tool and can be used to your advantage. Regularly practicing affirmative statements will help you

# RESTRUCTURING YOUR THOUGHTS

| EXAMPLE STRESSOR | HOW WOULD YOU REACT MENTALLY AND PHYSICALLY TO THIS STRESSOR? |
|---|---|
| You get cut off on the highway by another driver. | |
| You are at a restaurant, ready to leave, and it seems like you are waiting forever for the check. | |
| You need money at 8 P.M. and your card does not work at the ATM machine. | |
| You are walking to work from the train which was late, horns are blowing, construction crews are jackhammering, and a person running to catch the "walk" signal strongly bumps your shoulder as he goes by. He doesn't say "excuse me." | |
| Your friend or spouse is in the hospital. | |

FIGURE 6.6     Restructuring Your Thoughts

to keep things in perspective and set you at ease. Some commonly used statements are:

- "Is this really worth worrying about this much?"
- "Keep cool. Relax."
- "I can be miserable for a little while—then I will go have fun."
- "I do not have to be perfect. I can make mistakes. I do not have to please everyone."
- "It may feel like the end of the world, but I know I can cope."
- "Life often throws me curves; I will handle them."
- "I will keep this in perspective."
- "Not every argument is worth trying to win. I will back down from them on occasion."
- "I can solve this problem later."
- "I am O.K. I will get through this."

Which ones ring true for you? Pick one or two to practice over the next few days or create a few of your own.

Negative thoughts can erode your immune system, your self-esteem, and your ability to manage stress. Encouraging words, on the other hand, can enhance these areas. They are powerful tools that enable you to modify your response to stressors. Here are some additional perspective-altering ideas:

| Instead of thinking | Tell yourself |
|---|---|
| "I can't do this" | "I am confident; maybe I can" |
| "I'm nervous about this" | "I feel calm" |
| "I'm uptight about this" | "I don't have to worry" |
| "This is overwhelming" | "I am capable" |
| "I don't think I can do this" | "I can do this" |
| "This is not possible" | "I can find a way" |
| "I can't make these changes" | "I can probably make steady progress—one step at a time" |

Outlook and attitude play an extremely important role in whether or not life is stressful for you. As you learn to successfully focus your mind and shift your thoughts to avoid those that are self-defeating, you will find yourself managing your stress well. Healing the mind is as important as healing the body.

## Laugh—It's Good for You!

Everyone enjoys a good laugh, but you may want to laugh even more when you learn that there are both physical and mental benefits to be gained in the process. The physical benefits include achieving a state of relaxation (decreased heart rate, decreased blood pressure, decreased breathing rate, and decreased muscle tension). The mental benefits include an overall good feeling and distraction from negative thoughts. An added bonus of distraction is that it may buy you some extra time to calm down, relax, and look at a situation or event differently.

Humor can be used to your advantage for handling stress when it is well intentioned. However, when it is negative or offensive (using sarcasm or racial, sexist, and ethnic language), it is not a useful coping technique. Negative humor provides no lasting physical or mental benefits. Humor best promotes a sense of mental, emotional, and spiritual well-being when it is used kindly.

### What's So Funny?

We asked a group of recovering heart patients what makes them laugh and how they use humor therapy as a coping strategy. Here's what they had to say:

- You don't always have to smile—that's unrealistic. I go exploring for something fun to do when I'm feeling down.
- I don't take life too seriously. That's the ticket! Just take the time and make a conscious effort to live on the lighter side.
- I'm not one for joke telling. A lighthearted movie, TV program, or play works well for me.

- Have you ever seen a stand-up comedian? It's never too late.
- I pretend that I am Julia Child for the day in the kitchen and create the finest new recipe I can. Oh, what fun!
- Play with kids! They'll always keep you laughing.
- My friend Tammy always makes me laugh. When I need a mood change, I just call on her.
- Be creative. I find my humor in art, writing, and reading.
- I'm more of the imaginative type. I like to overexaggerate when I tell a story or joke.
- I've made a humor library at home that has videos, fun books, and funny tapes. When I feel a need for comic relief I go to my library and enjoy!
- I keep trying new things. I figure I've got nothing to lose.

The addition of humor to your life can change your perspective and your health. Use it as often as you can, laugh after laugh! The possibilities are endless. Whatever strategy you choose to introduce humor into your life, remember to keep it up on a regular basis. In reality, nothing is as important as we think it is in times of stress. A light attitude is the right attitude!

## Manage Your Environment

Balancing multiple roles in family, work, friendships, community, church, and other arenas can be quite a challenge. These multiple roles add to your cumulative stress. You cannot be everything to everyone at the same time. You have to make yourself and your health a number one priority. As you learn to gain perspective by restructuring your thoughts, these things will be easier to do:

- Take care of yourself as diligently as you would take care of others.
- Take on only what you are capable of handling comfortably.
- Be assertive. Express your needs and feelings.

- Manage your time efficiently. Use a day planner to budget both work and rest periods.
- Negotiate with others. Share roles and responsibilities.
- Say "no" when you need to. Realize you need down time.
- Let some things wait until tomorrow.
- Avoid the traps: "I have to . . ." "I can't . . ." "I should . . ." "I must . . ." "If only . . ."
- Be flexible. Make changes in your schedule to accommodate breaks for yourself.
- Delegate tasks to family members.
- Communicate expectations.
- Establish priorities.
- Make healthy decisions.

Existing in "high gear" all the time will exhaust you. Make sensible changes in your environment to reduce your stress buildup and add to your comfort level.


## Watch Out for the Traps

People often use stress as an excuse for practicing poor health habits such as drinking too much alcohol; smoking; consuming excessive amounts of caffeine, sugar, and sodium; and eating too much or too little. Practicing poor health habits may prolong stressful episodes.

- *Alcohol.* Although some research has found that an intake of 2 ounces or less of alcohol on a daily basis may reduce the risk of heart disease for some individuals, other studies have clearly shown that consuming more than 2 ounces of alcohol a day may contribute to high blood pressure. Additional research has found that prolonged and excessive drinking bouts (more than 4 ounces a day) can lead to health problems such as cirrhosis of the liver, heart disease, and certain cancers. It also can interfere with your relationships with family and friends and disrupt your sleep.

- *Smoking.* Smoking raises the heart rate and blood pressure, thereby mimicking a stress response. Adding to your stress unnecessarily will likely also increase your risk for future health problems. People who continue to smoke following a cardiac event greatly increase the risk that blockages will continue to develop in their arteries, which can lead to another heart attack.
- *Caffeine, sugar, and sodium.* Too much caffeine can make you feel irritable and interrupt sleep patterns. Too much sugar can cause extreme fluctuations in your body's sugar and energy levels, resulting in fatigue, irritability, and anxiety. Too much sodium can lead to problems such as high blood pressure.
- *Overeating/undereating.* Overeating can lead to obesity, and undereating can decrease your energy level and deplete vitamin stores. In either case, the long-term result of practicing poor dietary habits is future health problems.

These unhealthy ways of coping with stress are ineffective because, by using them, you avoid those healthy techniques that can help you identify and resolve the underlying cause of your stressors. They may offer temporary relief from distress but, in the long run, will make matters worse. To minimize your unhealthy reactions to stress, examine your dietary habits and find out why and when you eat and drink the things you do. You may be reacting to or avoiding something stressful. Eating well helps you to feel better and cope better, so decide what you need to change and do so gradually. Review chapter 5 for detailed information about managing your diet.

## Practice Healthful Habits

You can work out your stress in healthy ways by participating in regular exercise, getting adequate rest, and practicing relaxation techniques.

### *Exercise Regularly*

As you learned in chapter 4, when you are in good physical condition you are better able to resist stress. Regular exercise helps to strengthen your body, mind, and spirit. It improves the function of your heart, relaxes tense muscles, calms your body, and dissipates emotions such as depression, anxiety, and anger. You do not have to be athletic to exercise, nor do you have to participate in sports to gain the benefits exercise has to offer. What is important, however, is that you choose moderate-intensity activities you enjoy and that you will do on a regular basis.

As we discussed in chapter 4, stretching is considered an important part of your exercise program. When it comes to stress management, stretching is a useful coping strategy because it promotes a full-body relaxation response. The added bonus of stretching is that it can be done anywhere and at any time. Try stretching daily for ten to fifteen minutes in addition to your exercise program to relieve stress. Use the stretching examples provided in chapter 4 as your guide.

### *Get Adequate Rest*

Getting an adequate amount of rest will increase your productivity and efficiency, keep you on an even keel, and give you the energy you need to combat the daily stressors of life. Too much activity, long waking hours, and excess alcohol and caffeine can throw your natural sleep patterns out of balance. As a result of this imbalance, you may find yourself waking up suddenly in the middle of the night or very early in the morning only to toss and turn. If stress is affecting your sleep, try these comforting solutions:

1. Exercise earlier in the day rather than before sleeping. It can be hard to relax if you are active too close to bedtime.
2. Try drinking a glass of milk or eating a banana, which contain substances that help you to sleep.
3. Take a warm bath or shower before retiring and listen to your favorite calming music.

4. Plan at least two ten- to thirty-minute rest periods or naps during your day. Even if you just lie down but do not sleep, you are still helping to replenish your body's energy needs. Some people prefer just one nap period of sixty to ninety minutes. However, avoid naps if you find that they make nighttime sleep difficult.

### Practice Relaxation Techniques

Relaxation techniques are easy to learn and very beneficial for individuals recovering from a heart attack or bypass surgery. Relaxation techniques promote both physical and emotional benefits, including improved circulated oxygen to the heart, improved recovery from illness, and overall improved psychological adjustment. Responses to relaxation include decreases in heart rate, breathing rate, blood pressure, and muscle tension. As you begin to practice your relief strategies, consider both timing and the environment in which you choose to practice your favorite methods:

- When—on a regular basis. Daily practice is very beneficial.
- Where—in a comfortable and quiet environment.
- Position—sitting or lying down is preferable.
- How long—about ten to twenty minutes is desirable.
- Mind focus—concentration leads to success!

All are important contributors. No matter what method you choose, you will be able to stop a stress response before it stops you!

### Relaxation Technique #1: Relax Your Muscles

When your muscles are tense, progressive muscular relaxation can provide soothing relief. This relaxation technique is generally tried first because it is effective for almost everyone who tries it. Developed in the 1920s by Dr. Edmund Jacobson, progressive muscle relaxation is so named because you tense and then relax the muscles in the body from toe to head, relaxing more and more deeply as you go. The point of focus in this technique is the tension and then relaxation in your muscles.

Jacobson showed that you cannot relax your muscles and still worry at the same time. He also demonstrated that the brain becomes used to chronic muscle tension and that it takes an increase in muscle tension to jolt the brain's arousal center into relaxing unnecessary tension. In this technique, we purposefully tense our muscles, then deeply relax. As we concentrate on the contrast between tension and relaxation, we retrain our brains to recognize tension as it starts. This can greatly aid us in warding off tension headaches and backaches.

The instructions for this relaxation technique follow. You may read the script to yourself as you practice, have another person read the sequence to you, or place these instructions on an audio cassette. Before you begin, pay attention to position, temperature, and how restrictive your clothing is. Practice this technique while lying comfortably (arms at your sides with your palms facing upward) on a carpeted floor or seated (if you prefer). As your technique improves, you can try it just about anywhere.

---

**PROGRESSIVE MUSCLE RELAXATION SCRIPT:**

We are about to progressively tense and relax the major muscle groups in the body. This is a very effective way to reduce general arousal and muscle tension. I'll first explain the exercise for each area, and then ask you to tense by saying, "Ready? Tense." Tense relatively hard, but always stop short of discomfort or cramps. Tense until you are aware of tension in the area. Fully pay attention to it, and then study its contrast—relaxation. You'll tense for about five to ten seconds and then relax for about twice that long. For areas that are injured or sore, simply avoid tensing those areas or else tense very gently and slowly.

*continued*

To prepare, please loosen tight clothing. Remove glasses, contact lenses, or shoes if you wish. Lie down comfortably on a firm mattress or on the floor, with a small pillow under the head and another under the knees. Rest your arms at your sides and let your legs lie straight with your feet relaxed.

1. To begin, please let your eyes close. As you distract from visual stimuli, it is easier to notice the pleasant rhythms of your breathing. Just pay attention to your breathing. Breathe gently and peacefully, noticing a slight coolness in the air entering your nostrils on the in-breath and a slight warmth on the out-breath. Throughout this exercise, just breathe normally—slowly, rhythmically, abdominally.

2. When I say tense, I'd like you to point both of your feet and toes at the same time, leaving the legs relaxed. Notice the pulling sensation, or tension, in the calves and the bottoms of the feet. Form a clear mental picture of this tension. Now relax all at once. Feel the relaxation in those same areas. When muscles relax, they elongate, and blood flow through them increases. So you might feel warmth or tingling in areas of your body that you relax. Just let your feet sink into the floor, completely relaxed.

3. Next, pull your toes back toward your head. Ready? Tense. Observe the tension in the muscles below the knee, along the outside of the shins. Now relax all at once and see and feel the difference as those muscles fully relax and warm up.

4. Next, you'll tense the quadricep muscles on the front part of the leg above the knee by straightening your leg and locking your knees. Leave your feet relaxed. Ready? Tense. Concentrate on the pulling in these muscles. See it clearly in your mind. And relax. Scan your quadriceps as you relax. Sense them loosening and warming, as though they are melting.

5. Imagine now that you are lying on a beach blanket. Keeping your feet relaxed, imagine pressing the back of the heels into the sand. Ready? Tense. Feel and see the tension along the backs of the entire legs. Now relax as those muscles loosen and relax.

6.  A slightly different set of muscles, those between the upper legs, are tensed when you squeeze your knees together. Ready? Tense. Observe the tension. Then relax and observe the relaxation as you deeply relax, and keep relaxed, all the muscles in the legs as we progress upward. Just let the floor support your relaxed legs.

7.  Next, you'll squeeze the buttocks or seat muscles together while contracting your pelvic muscles between the legs. Leave your stomach relaxed as you do this. Ready? Tense. Visualize the tension in these muscles. Then relax and observe what relaxation in those muscles is like—perhaps a pleasant warm and heavy feeling.

8.  Next, you'll tense your stomach muscles by imagining your stomach is a ball and you want to squeeze it into a tiny ball. Ready? Tense. Shrink your stomach and pull it back toward the spine. Notice the tension there and how tensing these muscles interferes with breathing. Now relax. Let the abdomen warm up and loosen up, freeing your body to breathe in the least fatiguing way. Continue to breathe abdominally as you progress.

9.  Now leave your shoulders and buttocks down on the floor as you gently and slowly arch your back. As you do, pull your chest up and toward your chin. You'll observe the tension in the back muscles along both sides of the spine. Now gently and slowly relax as your back sinks into the floor, feeling very warm and relaxed. Study that feeling. Notice where relaxation is experienced.

10. Tense the lower back muscles by pressing the lower back against the floor. Ready? Tense. Observe the tension there, then relax and observe the relaxation in that area.

11. Prepare to press your shoulders downward, toward your feet, while you press your arms against the sides of your body. Ready? Tense. Feel the tension in the chest, along the sides of the trunk, and along the back of the arms. You may not have been aware of how much tension can be carried in the chest or what that feels like. Relax, and feel those muscles loosen and warm. Realize that you can

*continued*

control and release the tension in your upper body once you are aware of it.

12. Now, shrug your shoulders. Ready? Tense. Pull them up toward your ears and feel the tension above the collarbones and between the shoulder blades, where many headaches originate. Now relax and study the contrast in those muscles.

13. Place your palms down on the floor. Pull your relaxed hands back at the wrists so that the knuckles move back toward your head. Observe the tension on the top of the forearms. Relax and study the contrast.

14. Next, make tight fists and draw them back toward the shoulders as if pulling in the reins on a team of wild horses. See the tension in the fists, forearms, and biceps. Relax and notice the feelings as those muscles go limp and loose. Just let your arms fall back beside your body, palms up, heavy and limp and warm. Pause here to scan your body and notice how good it feels to give your muscles a break. Allow your entire body to remain relaxed as you move on.

15. Let's learn how to relax the neck muscles, which typically carry much tension. Right now, gradually, slowly turn your head to the right as if looking over your right shoulder. Take ten seconds or longer to rotate the neck. Feel the tension on the right side of the neck pulling your head around. The sensation on the left side is stretching, not tension. Hold the tension for awhile to observe it. Then turn around slowly back to the front and notice the difference as the muscles on the right side of your neck relax. Pause. Turn just as slowly to the left and watch the left side of your neck contract. Rotating back to the front, see the left side relax.

16. Now press the back of your head gently against the floor, while raising the chin toward the ceiling. Do you notice the tension at the base of the skull, where the skull meets the neck? Much headache pain originates here, too. Study the tension. And relax. Allow those muscles to warm up and elongate. Relax the neck all around and let it remain relaxed.

17. Lift your eyebrows up and furrow your brow. Feel the tension along the forehead. Relax. Imagine a rubber band loosening.

18. Wrinkle up your nose while you squeeze your eyes shut and your eyebrows together. Observe the tension along the sides of the nose, around and between the eyes. Now deeply relax those areas. Imagine pleasantly cool water washing over the eyes, relaxing them. Your eyelids are as light as a feather.

19. Frown, pulling the corners of the mouth down as far as they'll go. Feel the tension on the sides of the chin and neck. Relax. Feel the warm, deeply relaxing contrast.

20. The jaw muscles are extremely powerful and can carry much tension. When I say tense, clench your jaw. Ready? Tense. Grit your teeth and study the tension from the angle of the jaw all the way up to the temples. Observe the tension. Now relax and enjoy the contrast, realizing that you can control tension here, too. Relax the tongue and let the teeth part slightly.

21. Make a wide smile. Open the mouth wide. Ready? Tense. Grin ear to ear and feel the muscles around the cheekbone contract. This really requires little effort. Now relax and let all the muscles of the face now be smooth and completely relaxed. Allow a pleasant sense of relaxation to surround your body. Imagine that you are floating well supported on a favorite couch, bed or raft—all your muscles pleasantly relaxed. When you are ready to end this session, count slowly to five, send energy to your limbs, stretch, sit up slowly, and move your limbs before standing slowly.

Practice this twice a day for two weeks or more. At first you might be more aware of aches or tension in your muscles. This tends to disappear with practice as those tense muscles get a break and your nerves desensitize. With practice, you'll notice that you can relax your muscles passively, by just reminding yourself to relax them.

Source: Schiraldi, G. R. Conquer Anxiety, Worry and Nervous Fatigue: A Guide to a Greater Peace. Ellicott City, Md.: Chevron Publishing, 1997 (pp. 55–59). © 1997 Glenn R. Schiraldi. Reprinted with permission.

### Relaxation Technique #2: Take a Breather

Since your breathing becomes more shallow and rapid when you get excited during stress episodes, stopping this response quickly can help you to evaluate a situation more clearly and react more effectively. Breathing exercises provide instant relief because they can be done anywhere and at any time. One popular breathing technique, called diaphragmatic breathing, allows you to turn off your automatic breathing function and turn on your ability to control your breathing and your stress. Here's how it works. Simply find a comfortable position, focus your attention on your breathing, and follow the steps outlined below. Not only is this technique simple, it is also versatile. Once you've mastered the basics, try to combine this technique with other relaxation methods such as imagery (see relaxation technique # 3).

---

**DIAPHRAGMATIC BREATHING**
**("BELLY BREATHING")**

- Start by inhaling slowly through your nose and mouth. Feel the air go down into your lungs and stomach. Feel your stomach rise.
- Pause for a moment.
- Exhale slowly. Feel the air exit your stomach as it lowers. Feel the air continue to leave your lungs and leave your body.
- Repeat several times.

---

### Relaxation Technique #3: Picture a Pleasant Place

Using the power of your imagination is a great way to retreat from your stressors. These mental excursions typically involve a place, a scene, or an event that you remember as peaceful, restful, beautiful,

**IMAGERY EXERCISE**

- Sitting or lying down, close your eyes and take several slow, deep breaths.
- Picture yourself sitting comfortably at the beach.
- The sun is bright and its warmth feels wonderful as it touches your face, your arms, your chest, and your legs. Tell yourself you are relaxed. Picture yourself relaxed.
- The water touching your feet is cool and soothing.
- Feel the cool breeze from the ocean waves.
- Smell the freshness in the summer air.
- Today is a beautiful day. Not a cloud in the sky. You can see the water for miles.
- Listen to the waves splashing near the rocks. Relax.
- Take a deep breath through your nose and slowly exhale through your mouth.

and joyful. When you picture a pleasant place, try to engage all of your senses. For example, look for beauty, smell the fragrances, feel the air touch your skin, and listen to the sounds around you. This daydream technique helps your mind to reprogram itself, enabling you to relax at will, put things into perspective, and regain mental clarity and balance. Before you begin your mental escape, find a quiet place and assume a comfortable position. As you refine your imagery skills, take it on the road with you and use it to diffuse your next stressor. Try to master the approach by first using the example below, then be creative in discovering your own visual themes. For example, try creating a theme for healing your heart and a theme for making a health-conscious behavior change. Repeat these themes over and over in your mind until you believe them. Let them become a reality!

Other imagery suggestions:

- You are sitting by the fire on a snowy evening . . .
- You are lying under your warm covers in bed on a rainy Saturday morning . . .

### Relaxation Technique #4: Relaxing at Work

Do you often feel the pressure or tension building at work? Relief can be easily found if you make a few sensible changes in your daily routine.

### Relaxation Technique #5: Find Solitude

Relaxation can also result from focusing on your internal strength in a place of privacy. Visit a favorite place that is quiet. Your mind can be cleared of excess worries if you allow yourself to experience inner solitude. For example, your internal strength can be enhanced by meditating, writing in a journal, or participating in yoga.

## Find Support

One way to help you work through tense feelings is to build a support system. Share your feelings and concerns with the people who are important to you. Your relatives, friends, and co-workers are the people who make you feel good, who make your life easier, and on whom you rely in good times and bad. Supporters can listen to your concerns about important issues, including those that cause stress for you.

Use these people as a source of strength. Allow your support system to be a sounding board to vent your feelings, to provide feedback on your behavior, to assist you in changing your perspective, and to comfort you. Sometimes friends and family members are the first to notice a physical, emotional, and/or behavioral change that you exhibit. They can be an asset to your recovery.

Your ability to effectively cope with stress can be influenced by

## SUGGESTIONS FOR RELIEF AT WORK

- Schedule "interruptible" time. Take a laughter break regularly.
- Avoid noise, bad lighting, excessively cool or hot temperatures when you can. Adjust your environment so that it's comfortable at all times.
- Avoid overtime. Spend your evenings doing something you enjoy!
- Take a change-of-scenery break periodically. Walk away from your desk or outdoors.
- Take a "mental" break or a "fun" break to get lost in thought or to help you smile.
- Take a mental time-out before an important phone call, meeting, or presentation.
- Return phone calls before lunch or late in the workday when you will be less likely to get stuck talking longer than you would like.
- When your day gets difficult, STOP what you are doing and practice any one of the breathing exercises you just learned.

*Adapted from: Albrecht.* Stress and the Manager: Making It Work for You. *Englewood Cliffs, N.J.: Prentice-Hall, Inc., 1979.*

the number of social relationships you have, by the strength of these relationships, and by the lines of communication therein. What can you do to add to your social relationships? Can you try to develop new friendships and be more open with people? Share your thoughts and feelings about your stressors with your supporters, who can help you to more readily diffuse your stressors.

## Find a Spiritual Center

Finding a spiritual center and accepting your limitations can help you to reduce your stress and to heal. Not everyone is able to do this, but finding faith—whether it be in religion, nature, our own selves, or some other focus—can significantly help in your recovery and in managing your risk factors. Regardless of their origin, spiritual beliefs play powerful roles in our abilities to make positive changes in our lives. Living spiritually can help us to accept our limitations, move forward, reduce stress, and accept and love ourselves unconditionally.

Unconditional love, self-esteem, and stress management all relate to one another. To be able to accept, love, value, and respect one's self is paramount to your ability to successfully manage your stress. People with low levels of self-esteem often feel powerless, helpless, hopeless, and unable to meet new challenges; people with high levels of self-esteem generally feel enthusiastic about new challenges, capable of experiencing a wide range of emotions, and confident in their abilities. If you care about yourself, you will be able to take care of yourself! Use the strength your spiritual health can generate to maintain a high level of self-esteem, to make rational sense out of your illness, to accept your limitations, and to choose attitudes that will ultimately lead toward improved health behaviors. The power of the spirit is great!

## Putting Things in Perspective

The fact that you have heart disease may add to your emotional stressors. As we discussed in chapter 3, feelings of anxiety, depression, anger, denial, frustration, loss of confidence, worry, concern, and fear are common emotional stages through which recovering heart patients tend to progress. Experiencing these responses more often or in combination with other daily stressors can lead to unhealthy prolonged stress buildups.

**A NOTE TO FAMILY AND FRIENDS**

Stress management can be a family affair. Although you don't need to share all of the same coping strategies as your loved one, you can find some techniques that can be practiced together. Try taking a relaxation class together, becoming involved in couples massage therapy, or just taking the time to have fun with each other. This chapter can help you to see the warning signs of stress—both in yourself and your partner. By doing this, you will be helping your loved one and improving your own health at the same time.

Remember, our bodies are well equipped to deal with a reasonable amount of stress, even with heart disease. Remind yourself that the emotional impact of illness is only temporary and you can work through tense feelings. You can begin focusing your attention away from negative emotions and toward better health by examining the origin of these thoughts. As a result of turning your attention to wellness, you may progress through emotional turmoils more quickly and with less uncertainty.

**KICKING YOUR STRESS HABIT**

*Congratulations!* You have completed the third step in kicking your stress habit:

Step 3 = *learning additional coping strategies that you can adopt*

## STEP 4:
## HAVE A PLAN

To avoid getting stuck along the way, continually reevaluate how you think and respond to your stressors, restructure your thoughts when possible, and remind yourself of the endless possibilities for solutions.

### Know What to Do in a Crisis

If any physical or psychological symptoms continue or if you feel particularly "overwhelmed," contact your doctor. It is possible that your stress-related emotional symptoms (especially feelings of depression and/or low levels of self-esteem) have interfered with your ability to make healthy lifestyle changes. Your doctor may recommend resources such as stress management and relaxation programs often found in hospitals and community centers, or specialists who are well qualified to help you cope with your stressors. When it feels like a crisis is upon you, remember that you are not alone. Seek the support of family, friends, or a professional counselor. Hidden within each crisis is an opportunity for change, learning, and health gains just waiting to be discovered! (See Table 6.1.)

### Try Not to Overreact

Since you know stress can be induced by your reaction to a situation, realize that overreacting to little annoyances can cause unnecessary tensions. Remind yourself that you cannot always control what happens around you, but you can control how you respond. Life is filled with unexpected storms that will catch you off guard. The more flexible you are when a storm hits, the better equipped you will be to ride it out!

**TABLE 6.1     Solutions to Stressors**

| IF THIS IS YOUR PROBLEM . . . | HERE'S WHAT YOU CAN DO . . . |
|---|---|
| "I have heart disease and I am afraid to do anything." | **Change your perspective.** With proper management, you can live your life to the fullest extent of your abilities. Avoid adopting a grim outlook on life— it is only self-defeating. Strive to think positively. |
| "So much of my time is spent working long hours, tending to my family's needs, and planning for the future." | **Do something you enjoy.** There must always be time for you. |
| "Since my heart attack, all I do is count calories, watch my cholesterol and fat intake, and keep a regimented exercise schedule." | **Adopt a lighter attitude.** It does not have to be all work and no play. Discover the balance! |
| "I'm worried about getting well, but I don't want to unnecessarily burden my friends and family with my concerns." | **Find support.** Asking someone to help or simply to listen is OK. |

## Be Ready for Change

Stress is a reaction to change. You will find you will be more successful when you prepare yourself for change and progress slowly thereafter. Expect to feel uneasy at first as you attempt something new, such as changing the way you think and respond or adopting new coping strategies. Whenever you stray from your habits and try behaviors that are unfamiliar to you, you are bound to feel uncomfortable and vulnerable at times. So don't try to do too much too soon! Making changes can be hard, but if you take it slowly, step by step, you'll find that taking the risk of making a change was really worthwhile. Do it! You'll be glad you did.

## Set Goals

Setting goals will help you to manage lifestyle changes. Begin by setting small stress management goals first; then progress to larger stress management goals as each smaller goal is met. It is helpful to write down your goals and keep them in a visible location. Further, it is important to reevaluate them on occasion so that adjustments can be made to ensure success. See chapter 8 for more information on setting goals.

## Have a Plan

You will have greater success when you personalize your stress management program. Developing a stress management plan is simple. First, identify your stressors (big and small); second, prioritize stressors according to which you want to tackle first; third, identify when your stressors occur; and fourth, write your action plan for better managing your stress. Use Figure 6.7 to formulate your plan. Be as specific as possible. Refer to this plan regularly to monitor your progress. Keep it where you can refer back or add to it so that you can see what did or did not work when new stressors enter your life.

## MY STRESS MANAGEMENT PLAN

| MY STRESSORS ARE | PRIORITY # | IN WHAT SITUATIONS DOES MY STRESS OCCUR? | I PLAN TO . . . |
|---|---|---|---|
| Time management | 1 | Home/family chores | 1. Delegate cleaning responsibilities to my children. <br><br> 2. Evaluate time and effort for new work projects. |

FIGURE 6.7    Stress Management Worksheet

### KICKING YOUR STRESS HABIT

*Congratulations!* You have completed the fourth step in better managing your stress:

Step 4 = *having a plan*

## PUTTING IT ALL TOGETHER

Stress, left unmanaged, will increase your risk for future health problems. The challenge of stress management involves becoming aware of your prolonged and unrelenting stress episodes, recognizing what you can change, and learning to calm yourself quickly to reduce the negative impact stress can impose on your health. Making sensible lifestyle changes that include practicing your best coping strategies will assist you in meeting this challenge. Keep in mind that your success will largely depend on how you perceive and experience changes, not the actual number of changes you attempt or how quickly you achieve them. Coping is a process that occurs over time, not overnight!

To effectively manage your stress, slow down, reduce the tensions of daily living, learn to restructure your thoughts, practice relaxation techniques, adopt social skills that will give you more control, and monitor your progress throughout. Remember, managing your stress takes discipline, time, and effort. As you learn to evaluate the choices in your life and to identify your own coping style, you will accept the fact that stress is a necessary part of living, understand that your body is well-equipped to handle a reasonable amount of stress, and enjoy life's challenges along the way.

---

### KICKING YOUR STRESS HABIT

*Congratulations!* You have learned the "common threads" of stress management.

Step 1: *Recognize the warning signs of stress*
Step 2: *Identify coping strategies that you may already use*
Step 3: *Learn additional coping strategies that you might adopt*
Step 4: *Have a plan*

## REFER TO THIS LIST AS OFTEN AS NEEDED . . .

- Laugh it off
- Choose happiness
- Change your attitude
- Accept what is
- Develop hobbies
- Take a breather
- Think "I can"
- Have fun
- Be optimistic
- Do not rush
- Replace negatives with positives
- Visit a friend
- Talk less and listen more
- Don't doubt your abilities
- Take control
- Have a plan "B"
- Let yourself be happy
- Let go of things beyond your control
- Avoid negative people
- Be honest
- Learn to enjoy your life

- Say something nice
- Exercise regularly and eat right
- Make mistakes
- Anticipate when you need more time
- Smile
- Pace yourself
- Meditate
- Take time out
- Rest
- Learn to let go
- Avoid the quick fix
- Learn to relax
- Ask for help
- Keep a lighter attitude
- Make a choice
- Delegate
- Join a support group
- Seek new adventures
- Set priorities
- Count backward slowly from 10 to 1

*continued*

- Don't be a perfectionist
- Listen to music
- Avoid procrastination
- Take a long bath or a hot shower
- Watch your drinking
- Accept gracefully
- Don't worry
- Read a book
- Reduce uncertainty
- Ask for clarification
- Negotiate
- Take a deep breath
- Know where to turn
- Take the time now
- Develop interests
- View troubles as opportunities
- Don't make excuses
- Speak up
- Plan
- Enjoy your leisure time
- Be understanding
- Eliminate irrational thinking

- Cooperate
- Plan a vacation
- Minimize the problem
- Anticipate
- Put things in  perspective
- Welcome change
- Be assertive
- Get a massage
- Enjoy the company of a pet
- Retreat to a spa
- Believe in yourself
- Make your favorite meal
- Reward yourself
- Avoid noise
- Try not to overreact
- Pause before responding
- Write in your journal
- Play with a child
- Slow down
- Recall an unforgettable sight
- Awaken to classical music
- Live spiritually

§

## CHAPTER SEVEN

# SEEKING A
# HEALTHY BALANCE

ACHIEVING BALANCE DEPENDS ON COMMITMENT. YOU NEED TO recognize the limits of your illness in order to safely enjoy the freedoms of an active lifestyle. Commitment and balance can be gained by actively participating in your care and taking precautions that will ensure your safety at all times.

This chapter will help you strike the right balance between being complacent about your health care and becoming actively involved in your recovery. We will explore the role of the health care team and strategies to developing positive relationships. We will tell you how to take advantage of educational resources that will enable you to better understand heart disease and how to interpret and critique health information presented in the media. We will help you understand how to properly use medications to maximize their potential and reduce side effects. Finally, you will learn how to balance safety and adventure by practicing preventive measures meant to let you safely take part in outdoor activities.

## PARTICIPATE IN YOUR PROGRESS

Actively participating in your own progress begins with an understanding that you are the captain of a team who will assist you during your recovery and when you are well again. Each member of your team will accept a certain degree of responsibility for your health and help you establish health goals and make treatment decisions.

The members of your team may include any of the following professionals: a primary care doctor, a cardiologist, a surgeon, a clinical nurse specialist and/or nurse practitioner, and other health care providers (dietitians, physical and/or occupational therapists, physician assistants, exercise physiologists, social workers, and/or mental health professionals). Your supporters (family, friends, clergy, and so on) are members of your team as well. All these people will provide care, information, education, and advice.

Each member of your team has a specific talent and, therefore, a specific responsibility related to your successful recovery. Each one will also have a unique level of understanding about your illness and your goals for recovery. To be sure you receive quality care, do not assume that all team players are aware of all aspects of your treatment plan; often that is not the case. The better you understand your illness and the more confident you become about assuming your responsibilities and holding others accountable for theirs, the closer you will be to striking the right balance.

### Your Responsibilities

Your responsibilities include monitoring your day-to-day health and reporting any changes in how you feel to your doctor (especially new-onset or changing symptoms, sudden weight changes, decreased ability to perform a particular activity, and/or side effects to medications). You also must take your prescribed medications exactly as your doctor has advised. Finally, you must follow any specific recommendations your doctor makes, including a special diet plan and/or guidelines for social activities, exercise, and work.

Following through on your end of the bargain is only a part of the process. To strike the right balance and feel satisfied with your care, you will need to take it a step further. You must become an active participant in your own progress by verbalizing questions and concerns about your recovery plan. You can start by finding a doctor you like and trust. This will help you to be more comfortable about visiting the doctor's office, asking questions, and communicating directly about your concerns.

### Find a Doctor You Like and Trust

Finding a doctor you like and trust can mean the difference between receiving adequate or excellent care, and feeling dissatisfied or satisfied with your progress. Because the doctor-patient relationship is unique, it is important that you take the time to find the right match. Think about these general considerations when you are searching for a doctor. First, try to match your doctor's qualifications with your needs. Knowing that your doctor is an expert in an area that is important to you will make you more confident in his or her ability to give you the best possible care. Second, try to match the doctor's approach to treatment with yours. Finally, look for personality traits that match yours. For example, are you more comfortable with a doctor who is respectful, direct, courteous, and/or listens well? Just as some friends "click" and others do not, the same holds true for you and your doctor. How well you get along with your doctor is important and will affect how comfortable you are at office visits, how well you communicate, and how likely you are to follow his or her advice.

### Be Relaxed at the Doctor's Office

It is not unusual for individuals to feel anxious, embarrassed, and timid when visiting a doctor's office. There can be lots of reasons for these feelings, but often they come from a lack of understanding about heart disease or illness, an inability to communicate effectively with health care providers, and an unfamiliarity with health care environments and procedures. To reduce these awkward feelings at the doctor's office, talk to your doctor and share your concerns. Discuss your fears, how well you understand what he or she is saying, and your comfort level regarding how he or she is managing your care.

As the two of you get to know one another, your visits will go more smoothly. As office visits become more comfortable, you may also find that speaking confidently and openly and asking questions will come easier as well.

### *Ask Questions and Be Prepared for Your Office Visits*

All questions are good questions and are worth asking. Getting answers to your questions will help you to improve your understanding of heart disease, raise your confidence in managing your care, and increase your overall level of satisfaction. Consider the following practices with regard to questioning and visiting your doctor:

- Write down your questions at home as you think of them. Sometimes you may think of a question after a doctor visit. Write it down for your next visit (unless it is extremely urgent).
- Arrive at your doctor's office with your list of questions. Some people find it helpful to write down the doctor's answers during the visit so that they can reread them later. You may feel more confident leaving the doctor's office with your answers in hand.
- Make the most of your time and try not to get sidetracked. Talk about things that directly relate to your care.
- Be sure that you understand any instructions (for example, details about your medication schedule, diet, or activity restrictions) before you leave the office. Clarify anything about which you are uncertain.
- If you are visiting your doctor because of a change in your clinical condition, bring a written description of your problems. Be as specific as possible when you describe recent illnesses or symptoms.

- Talk over your treatment options with your doctor and others involved. Feel free to get a second opinion.
- Talk about your expectations. Misunderstood expectations can quickly lead to dissatisfaction and disappointment.
- Bring someone along for support to your office visits. Two heads are better than one, and it is comforting to know you can talk about your office visit, treatment options, and instructions with someone who can understand.
- If for any reason you change doctors or have another doctor added to your team, be prepared to provide this person with a clear summary of your illness, present medical symptoms, past medical history, medications, and social history. This will help to ease the transition for this new team member.

What questions should you ask your doctor? Some of the questions you will want to ask your doctor or other health providers will be obvious. Others won't. This is typically the case if you haven't had much experience with doctors. Below are some important questions that you should be ready to ask your doctor:

1. What is the best way to reach you?
2. What are the signs and symptoms that I am getting worse?
3. What complications might occur during my recovery?
4. What side effects are common with the medications I am taking?
5. What should I do if I have any side effects from medications?
6. Will the nonprescription drugs I take interfere with my prescription medicines?
7. How will I know when I am making progress?
8. Are my goals realistic?

Next time you visit your doctor, be prepared for the questions he or she may ask you and be ready to ask your own questions in addition to those listed above. This will help you get over the overwhelming feeling that often accompanies uncertainty. It also will be helpful to arrive at your doctor's office with the intention of being an active participant in all discussions.

### Be Direct About Your Concerns

If you are actively involved in your medical care, speak your mind, and make decisions, you will be more likely to get better care and end up healthier than if you are passive. You can improve your skills in these areas if you learn as much as you can about your illness and how to live with it from knowledgeable individuals and reliable resources. We will address these important points throughout this chapter.

Since your demeanor at the doctor's office can influence the type of care you receive, try not to be too pushy with the demands you place on your doctor. To strike the right balance, do not rush to or call your doctor's office for the "small stuff." Try to manage your minor health problems at home. Discovering the balance also involves having a give-and-take relationship with your doctor. You need to be both assertive and flexible.

### Gaining Satisfaction

Now that you understand the kind of relationship you want with your doctor, how to find a doctor you like and trust, how to feel more comfortable at the doctor's office, and how to communicate directly about your concerns, you will also find that you are more satisfied with your overall care. Try to be friendly with your doctor and with other health professionals that work on your recovery team. These relationships will help motivate you to follow instructions and guide you through a full recovery.

## Your Doctor's Responsibilities

Your doctor's responsibilities include giving you the best possible care, prescribing the right medications, listening to your concerns, allowing time for your questions, talking to you in a way you can clearly understand, and treating you equitably, with respect, and with courtesy.

## Your Family's Responsibilities

Include your family in your care and in your progress. Family members need to learn with you. They need to understand your illness, seek health information with you, make adjustments in their lifestyles that will complement yours, and feel that they are a part of your recovery team. They, too, will be living with your heart disease. Rely on your family for support and to lighten your load, but don't let family members assume responsibility for your health.

Strong family members can provide a source of support for you, help you monitor your day-to-day health, help you understand symptoms that are both typical and unusual for you, and recognize when they should intervene in reporting changes in your health condition directly to your health care providers when you don't do so yourself. Your family should also be prepared for questions a health care provider may commonly ask:

1. What is the patient being treated for?
2. What are the names, doses, and frequency of the patient's medications?
3. Was a medication dose(s) missed?
4. Did the patient take all medications as prescribed?
5. Describe the patient's symptoms. Be as specific as possible. Know the problem/complaint, location, degree of discomfort, duration of discomfort, any worsening of the problem over time, any accompanying symptoms, whether the symptom was induced with exertion or not, and whether the symptom is new or different in nature.
6. Has the patient done anything to relieve/resolve his/her symptom?

**STRIKING THE RIGHT BALANCE:**
**THE TEAM APPROACH**

- You can gain more information and better control of your health if you become an active participant in managing your care. Become a team player.
- *Your responsibilities* include monitoring your day-to-day health, following specific instructions and guidelines that your health care providers suggest, reporting changes in how you feel to your doctor immediately, and becoming an active participant in your progress.
- *Your doctor's responsibilities* include providing the best possible care for you, communicating effectively with you, and treating you with respect and courtesy.
- *Your family's responsibilities* include providing support and actively involving themselves in your care.

## SEEKING INFORMATION

In order to improve your effectiveness in participating in your progress and in better managing your care, you will need to educate yourself about your illness and the best strategies to ensure both good health and an improved quality of life. This does not mean that you have to read everything or believe everything you read. This section will help you to be choosy about what you read and what you believe. We will highlight how to select educational resources that will help you understand your illness and teach you how to evaluate sources of public health information.

Today, we know much more about heart disease and living with it than ever before. Each decade has brought new insights and medical breakthroughs in the treatment and clinical management of heart disease. For people living with this problem, these milestones have resulted in both improved health and longer life. As we learn more, we will be better able to prevent the progression of heart disease and improve the quality of life for people like you who are living with it.

Keeping up with medical breakthroughs and new information, however, can be challenging. There is an abundance of health information resources from which to choose. Your challenge will be to find the best of these resources. You have already taken the first step by choosing to read this book. This is a good beginning.

Your next step will be getting assistance from those who can help you progress in understanding the nature of heart disease: your doctor, your family and friends, and other resources. Appendix A will give you a valuable point of reference for seeking additional health information. Although this appendix is not all inclusive, it will provide you with a strong foundation of quality health education resources: associations and organizations, government agencies, library resources, and Internet resources, among others. As you begin to use these materials, you may find others that are worth adding to your resource list.

## BRIDGING THE COMMUNICATION GAP

In addition to these resources and the valuable information your doctor and other health professionals may provide, you also will be exposed to a great deal of health information on a daily basis from newspapers, journals, television, and magazine sources. This information is often presented in a complex manner and with conflicting viewpoints which make it difficult to assess its validity. Since this information can influence your thoughts and your behaviors, it is important that you understand the disparities between mass media and public health objectives so that you can evaluate science news stories more effectively.

Mass media objectives may include entertaining, making a profit, persuading, sharing significant findings, examining personal concerns, reporting popular topics, and reflecting societal values. Public health objectives, on the other hand, generally include educating, communicating complex information, addressing societal concerns, and improving public health. Because of these differences, you may find it both difficult and frustrating to interpret and understand health information. To help bridge this gap, we will review some important facts about how best to evaluate health information that is media driven.

## How to Evaluate Science News Stories

1. *Be skeptical of stories reported on TV and radio.* Because of time limitations, these stories often must be condensed, making it impossible to present important details. Look for more detail in the newspaper or a news magazine.
2. *Read headlines skeptically.* They are designed to attract attention and may be inaccurate or incomplete because they do not convey important details.
3. *Analyze the entire article.* Look to see where the research was done. Generally, the most credible research is done in large academic institutions, such as well-known medical schools or the National Institutes of Health (which includes such subsidiaries as the National Heart, Lung, and Blood Institute, the National Cancer Institute, and others). The U.S. Department of Agriculture also conducts some research. Also, look to see who the researchers are. Scrutinize their credentials and organizational affiliations. Finally, look to see if the research was published in a scientific journal or presented at a meeting. Usually studies published in a journal are reviewed by other scientists before publication and are more complete than those presented at meetings. Studies that are works in progress may

be presented at meetings so that the researcher can get feedback from other scientists.

4. *Check to see if the study was done with animals or humans.* Research from animal studies cannot be applied directly to humans. However, animal studies are often used to design human studies to research the same question. Likewise, the results of one study done with humans cannot be safely translated into recommendations for all humans. One study is only one link in a long chain of studies that must be done before reliable conclusions can be drawn.

5. *Note the age, gender, race, and other characteristics (such as socioeconomic status) of the subjects studied.* The results of the study should only be applied to similar populations and only if other studies confirm the results.

6. *Note the size of the population studied.* Theoretically, the larger the number being studied, the better—the results are more significant.

7. *Be skeptical of results reported only in percentages.* The absolute numbers should be given because they help to put things in proper perspective.

8. *Be cautious—don't jump to conclusions.* News reporting is competitive; there is pressure to report whatever is new. A bias against conventional wisdom may sometimes exist because what is commonly known is not newsworthy. Look at trends rather than single studies. Even in the research community, there may be pressure to announce results early. Preliminary results may be released early due to scientific competition, as a way to develop continuing financial support. It is important to remember that these results are not final. With more time and study, conclusions could change. Good science is slow; it may take years before a particular question is settled. Until final conclusions can be reached, contradictory studies may be reported. Do not be alarmed by controversy; this is a normal part of the

scientific process. Good researchers often review the same data and reach different conclusions. This is beneficial because debate raises more questions that require further study.

9. *Check with others.* Before acting on the results of any science news story, consult a qualified professional such as your doctor, a dietitian if the study relates to nutrition, or a nurse. The American Heart Association has a great deal of information about cardiovascular disease available for the public.

In addition to these important points, many research institutions have information available; the National Library of Medicine has public information available on the Internet, and there are both public information phone numbers and Web sites for each of the constituent institutes of the National Institutes of Health (one of the nation's foremost biomedical research centers).

The acquisition of new knowledge will affect your future health status, keep you informed, and will help you to make wise decisions about your future. Take the time to understand public health information, be selective in your readings, and evaluate all sources closely. Never change your treatment plan because of something you read, saw, or heard about without discussing it with your doctor first.

---

**STRIKING THE RIGHT BALANCE:**
**BRIDGING THE COMMUNICATION GAP**

- Mass communications may present health information in a complex manner and with conflicting viewpoints.
- Remind yourself of the disparities that exist between mass media and public health objectives.
- To bridge this communication gap, learn the facts about how to best evaluate health information and select your health information resources wisely.

## MEDICATION USE AND PRECAUTIONS

For many people, recovering from heart disease is managed by making lifestyle changes and adopting new health habits, as we have discussed in previous chapters. Medications can be used as an adjunct to lifestyle changes for the treatment of heart disease. They can help to prevent, shorten, and cure illness. When used properly, medications also can help you to lead a normal and productive life.

Before we discuss medication use, we will give you some background information about cardiac medications and the common therapeutic options from which your doctor may choose. Cardiac medications may be prescribed for a number of reasons, including:

1. *Angina.* Chest pain or pressure, sometimes felt in the arm, jaw, back, or upper abdominal areas, due to decreased blood supply to some portion(s) of the heart muscle. It is often precipitated by exertion, emotional stress, and/or cold exposure.
2. *Hyperlipidemia.* High serum cholesterol and/or high triglycerides.
3. *Hypertension.* High blood pressure.
4. *Congestive heart failure (CHF).* Fluid retention in the lungs, legs, and/or abdomen due to inadequate pumping ability of the heart or to severe narrowing or leaking of heart valve(s).
5. *Arrhythmias.* Rhythm disturbances of the heart.
6. *Coagulation.* Thickening of the blood.

There are a number of supportive medications used to treat these problems. It is important for you to become familiar with these medications and learn how they function in your body to keep your condition stable. Here are some of these options:

- *Nitrates.* These are an extremely effective group of medicines that help the heart receive more oxygen-rich blood, relieve most episodes of angina, and reduce the workload on the heart. This medication works by relaxing the veins and arteries.

- *Beta blockers.* These medicines keep your heart from beating too fast. They reduce heart muscle oxygen demands, blood pressure, and anginal episodes. These medications work by blocking structures in the body called beta receptors that normally function to stimulate the heart. They tend to be most effective within the first three years after a heart attack. They have been found to reduce both the reoccurrence of heart attacks and premature death after a heart attack.

- *Antiarrythmics.* These medications can help to prevent or correct heart rhythm irregularities. They work by reducing the excitability of the heart cells and by slowing the heart's electrical conduction system.

- *Aspirin and anticoagulant drugs.* These two families of medications help to prevent clots (which can cause a heart attack) from forming in the blood vessels. They are commonly referred to as "blood thinners." These medications work by inhibiting the clotting action of platelets (the smallest cells in the blood).

- *Cholesterol-lowering drugs.* These medications can help to lower total serum cholesterol, low-density lipoproteins (LDL), and triglyceride levels. Cholesterol medication can act in the intestine to prevent dietary intake from being absorbed, can act in the liver to prevent the formation of cholesterol in the liver, or can interfere with the body's processing of cholesterol.

- *Calcium channel blockers.* These medications help the muscles of the heart and blood vessels to relax, causing the blood pressure to be reduced. This relaxed state of the vessels decreases the likelihood that a spasm (twitching or involuntary contraction) will occur. These medications work by blocking calcium (the nutrient that causes the heart and blood vessels to contract).

- *ACE inhibitors.* These medications widen your blood vessels, making it easier for the heart to pump by strengthening each heartbeat. As a result, more blood can be pumped through the body. These medicines typically function to lower blood pressure and treat heart failure. They work by preventing the narrowing of blood vessels.

- *Digitalis.* This medication helps your heart to beat more effectively, with increased force, and to help stabilize heart rhythm irregularities. It works by slowing the heart's electrical system.
- *Diuretics.* These medications help to remove excess water and salt from the body that may otherwise accumulate in your ankles, feet, legs, and/or abdomen. Excess fluid retention can lead to high blood pressure and heart failure. Diuretics are commonly referred to as "water pills." These medications work by making you urinate more frequently and by blocking some of the body's reabsorption of salt. Often a potassium supplement is prescribed in conjunction with a diuretic medication because some diuretics cause the body to lose potassium.

How much and what type of medication your doctor prescribes will largely depend on the symptoms of your illness and the severity of your disease. Your responsibility is to take the proper dose of your medications at their specified times, follow exact guidelines for handling and storing medications, take precautions when traveling, and keep track of your medications.

## Using Your Medications Properly

If you follow your doctor's precise instructions you will find that cardiac medications can be used with ease. We will outline strategies to ensure proper use and to avoid the consequences of misuse.

### What happens if I abruptly stop taking my medications?
Severe hypertension, chest pain, including heart attack, and worsening of rhythm disturbances can occur when certain medications are suddenly stopped. Consult your doctor before discontinuing any cardiac medications. To avoid mishaps, do not wait until you run out before refilling your prescriptions.

### What happens if I miss a dose of my medicine?

The effects of missing an individual dose depend on the specific situation. In some cases, missing one dose is not harmful, but your schedule should be maintained as closely as possible in order to keep your heart rhythm stable, to prevent rises in your blood pressure, to prevent angina, and/or to maintain adequate blood clotting ability. Try not to get into the habit of missing medication doses or not filling your prescriptions in a timely manner, as the benefits of the medication can be reduced or lost completely. Do not take two doses if you forget one.

### How do my medications affect my ability to exercise?

Many people are able to exercise longer before the onset of angina when taking medications, including beta blockers, long-acting nitroglycerin, and calcium channel blockers. Often, people are able to do more at home and pursue recreational activities with minimal or no chest pain. As you begin to feel better, your doctor may reduce the dose or instruct you to discontinue the medication. Although medication adjustments may likely occur, you should never adjust your medication doses yourself.

### Does every medication have side effects?

All medications can potentially have side effects or unplanned results in addition to their intended effects. Some are bothersome, but not serious (for example, nausea or diarrhea), and others are potentially harmful (for example, fever, rash, low blood pressure, heart failure, or worsening of the heart rhythm). While some side effects can be dealt with by decreasing the dose of the medication, others require a change in the type of medication prescribed for you. Your doctor may choose a different medicine in the same family that works just as well but does not produce the unwelcome side effects. In other cases, your doctor may prescribe an additional medication specifically to treat your side effects. However your doctor chooses to manage your side effects, you should never take additional medications to treat side effects without your doctor's approval. Always report all side effects to your doctor immediately.

### Can medications have harmful effects?
Medications can have harmful effects. In some cases they can have a toxic (poisoning) effect if not taken as prescribed. For most medications, more is rarely better. In fact, for some people, increasing the dose of medication may be quite harmful. Always follow your doctor's precise instructions.

In other cases, medications can be potentially harmful if you are allergic to them (for example, sulfites or yellow dye). Be sure to inform your doctor of all your known allergies (to drugs, foods, or other substances) before taking any medications.

Finally, the use of any medication during pregnancy must be carefully evaluated. Certain medications may cause birth defects in your unborn baby. Other medications simply have not been determined to be safe for individuals who are pregnant.

### Why do people need different doses of medications?
First, whether you take medicine orally (by mouth), sublingually (under the tongue), or topically (on the skin), the absorption rate varies from individual to individual. The absorption rate is how fast your body begins to use the medicine. Thus, the dose will vary for different people. Second, the way that your body processes each medication will vary as well; some individuals will require more of the medicine in their bloodstreams and tissues than others to achieve the desired effect. It may take several weeks for your doctor to find the best dosage and combination of medicines for you. Be patient. The end result is worth waiting for. Once your doctor determines the right dosage and frequency combination, you will receive the maximal effect of the medication. Because absorption rates and the way your body processes medications vary from person to person, you should never take another individual's medication or give another person yours.

## *How do medications interact?*

Some medications combine well with others, and some do not. Your doctor will make sure that the combination of medications he or she prescribes will not place your health in jeopardy. It is important, however, that you keep a current written list of all your medicines with you at all times. This is particularly important if you have more than one doctor on your recovery team. It is possible that medications prescribed for one clinical condition may not fit well with medications that are prescribed for another. This even includes the use of nonprescription medications such as aspirin, cold remedies, and antacids. The doctors who are treating you for different problems will need to communicate with one another to determine the best medication schedule for you. Do not use additional drugs (including nonprescription ones) without obtaining your doctor's approval. In addition, you should ask your doctor or pharmacist if you may use alcohol with the medications you are taking. Often, the use of alcohol is discouraged.

## *What should I do if I take too much medication by mistake?*

If you think you took too much medication by mistake, call your doctor and/or the poison control center immediately. Both of these telephone numbers should be readily available by your telephone. In some instances, you may be told to take ipecac syrup, a substance that induces vomiting in an emergency situation.

## *What should I know about each medication I am taking?*

- What the medication is used for and how it may make you feel.
- The generic and brand name of the medication.
- Possible side effects of the medication.
- Your medication schedule: dose, frequency, and how to take.
- Any activity restrictions you have while taking this medication.

## STRIKING THE RIGHT BALANCE:
### USE MEDICATIONS WISELY

- Never stop taking your medication abruptly.
- Do not wait until you have run out of a medication before getting a refill of your prescription.
- Do not take two doses if you forget one.
- Never adjust your medication dosage yourself.
- Do not use additional medications (including nonprescription ones) without first obtaining your doctor's approval.
- Before using any medication, inform your doctor if you are pregnant and if you have ever had an allergic reaction to another medication.
- Never take someone else's medication or give them yours.
- If you are being treated for more than one clinical condition, be sure that all your doctors are aware of your medication schedule.
- Before using a medication, check to see that the container has not been tampered with or damaged. If this is the case, do not use this medication and refill your prescription immediately.
- Never take additional medications to treat side effects without first obtaining your doctor's approval.
- Always follow your doctor's precise instructions. If you feel a medication is not working for you, let your doctor know.

## Handling and Storing Your Medications

Handling and storing your medications is simple. Here are some practical tips to ensure medication effectiveness:

- Be sure that all your medicines are properly labeled. Each should include your pharmacy's name, address, and phone number; your name, prescription number, and doctor; instructions for usage; quantity, refill information, and date of expiration; and any special storage instructions. This is particularly important if anyone ever has to assist you in taking your medicines for any reason. Discard all outdated medications.

- Carry all medicines in their original containers. Transferring medicines from their original containers may decrease their potency or effectiveness and increase the possibility of taking the wrong one.

- Store medications in a cool, dry place. An area of low humidity and consistent temperature is best. Avoid storing medications in places like your pocket, your bathroom, a windowsill, your car glove compartment, or anywhere else where they can get hot or will be in direct sunlight. Heat and moisture can cause medications to break down and become less effective. Do not store medications in the refrigerator unless you have been instructed to do so.

## Taking Precautions When Traveling

Precautions should also be taken when traveling. Here are some practical tips to ensure safe travel:

- Carry a list in your wallet of your medicines (with notations of both generic and trade names) and a brief summary of your medical history (for example, a list of significant illnesses), allergies, and your doctors' names and phone numbers. It is also helpful to carry a reduced-size copy of your most recent electrocardiogram (picture of your heart rhythm).

- Take an ample supply of your medications with you. It is a good idea to have an extra prescription for your medicines in your wallet just in case you run out, especially if you are traveling out of the state or the country.
- Carry all medicines in their original containers in a carry-on bag. You never know when your baggage may be lost in transit.
- Do not combine different medications in the same container to save space. In the event that you may need assistance taking your medications, no one would know how to help you.
- Be sure to know how to seek medical assistance when you have arrived at your destination, particularly if you are traveling abroad.
- Take with you any food substitutes you may need. Airlines are happy to provide special meals (low fat, low sodium, low cholesterol, and so on) if notified at least twenty-four hours in advance. Ask about this when booking your flight.

## Keeping Track of Your Medications

To avoid making mistakes, it is best to keep a record of your medicines so that you know exactly which medications to take each day, what the dose is, what your medication looks like, what time of day and how your medication should be taken, and what your medication is used for. The medication record in Figure 7.1 will help you in this process. Keep a current copy of this record in your wallet at all times. In the event of an emergency, this information can be very helpful to health professionals who may be assisting you. As you use your medication record, try to establish a system or a regular practice that will ensure compliance in medication taking and prevent careless mishaps.

While there are some general rules to follow, the process can be simplified by learning about the medications being used to treat your illness and by taking all of them precisely as your doctor advises. When precautions such as proper handling and storing of

## MEDICATION RECORD

| NAME | DOSE | WHEN/HOW TO TAKE | SIZE, SHAPE, OR COLOR | USED FOR |
|------|------|------------------|-----------------------|----------|
| Lopressor | 50 mg | twice daily (with meals) | pink | high blood pressure, angina |

FIGURE 7.1    Sample Medication Record

your medications, being prepared for travel, and maintaining a written record of your medicines are taken, you will gain the maximal benefits your medications can provide for you.

## BALANCING SAFETY AND ADVENTURE

Factors such as temperature, air quality, altitude, and varied terrain can affect how you feel and how safely you exercise. When appropriate precautions are taken, however, you may find that your tolerance for outdoor exercise may improve and the times you feel distressed may be fewer.

## Temperature

Your body responds differently to hot and cold temperatures. In hot weather, your body temperature rises more rapidly. The blood is brought to the skin in order to reduce the body temperature by sweating. If too much water is lost through sweating, dehydration and a drop in blood pressure may occur. Table 7.1 describes some general practices to prevent this situation.

**TABLE 7.1     When the Weather Is Hot Outdoors . . .**

| DO'S | DON'TS |
|---|---|
| Drink plenty of water before, during, and after exercise. | Exercise outside if the temperature is over 80 degrees Fahrenheit. |
| Exercise during the cooler morning or evening hours when the temperature is below 80 degrees Fahrenheit with low humidity. | Use salt tablets. |
| Wear light colored cotton or cotton-blend clothes that are loose fitting. | Increase the intensity and/or duration of your exercise in warm weather. |
| Watch for symptoms of heat stress: dizziness, headache, nausea, irregular heartbeat, and/or cramps. If these symptoms occur, stop exercising, go indoors, drink plenty of cool liquids, and rest. If the symptoms are not relieved, seek medical attention immediately. | Exercise shortly after eating a meal. |
| Use sunscreen and a hat to keep the sun off your head. | Exercise if you feel uncomfortable exercising in warmer temperatures. |

During cooler weather, the body heat produced by exercise is transferred away from the body faster than it can be replaced. This may cause difficulty breathing, a faster heart rate and higher blood pressure, and an increased chance of angina. Follow the suggestions in Table 7.2 to prevent this situation.

**TABLE 7.2   When the Weather Is Cool Outdoors . . .**

| DO'S | DON'TS |
| --- | --- |
| Dress in layers. They create a natural insulation by trapping heat. | Exercise outdoors if the temperature is under 40 degrees Fahrenheit. Wait for the warmer part of the day to exercise. |
| Wear a wool hat, socks, gloves, and sweater. Wool provides warmth even when it is wet. | Increase the intensity and/or duration of your exercise in cold weather. |
| Wear a loose scarf around your nose and mouth to warm the air you breathe. | Exercise if you feel uncomfortable exercising in cooler temperatures. |

Talk to your doctor to see if snow shoveling is safe for you. If you live in an area where it snows regularly, consider hiring someone to remove the snow from your sidewalks or driveway, or use a power snowblowing device (with your doctor's approval). However, if you must move snow by hand, check with your doctor to be certain it will not put too much stress on your heart. Shoveling snow increases your heart rate, blood pressure, and your heart's demand for oxygen, and therefore should be done with caution. With your doctor's consent, snow shoveling can be done safely by following the general guidelines in Table 7.3.

**TABLE 7.3    Snow Shoveling Guidelines**

| DO'S | DON'TS |
|---|---|
| Move snow (if you must) only with your doctor's approval. | Move snow *without* your doctor's approval. |
| Inform a family member of your plans to shovel snow. | Hold your breath as you lift. Always exhale as you lift. |
| Warm up and stretch for ten minutes before starting. | Allow yourself to get out of breath. |
| Use a small lightweight shovel. Lift small amounts of snow at one time. Work in layers. Move the top level of snow first. Use your legs to help push the snow. | Continue shoveling if chest pain or discomfort occurs. It is best to stop your activity, go inside, and rest. Take NTG as prescribed by your doctor. Do not resume any strenuous activity on that day. Check with your doctor prior to performing this activity again. |
| Dress warmly in layered clothing. | Consider snow shoveling part of your exercise program. |
| Shovel in ten-minute periods. Take frequent breaks. | Consume alcohol before, during, or immediately after shoveling. |

Whether you are moving snow or walking in warm weather, you need to be aware of atmospheric conditions in addition to temperature considerations.

## Air Quality

Exercise makes everyone more vulnerable to health complications from polluted air because the amount of air taken in can increase by as much as ten times the level at rest. For persons with heart disease, poor air quality may cause angina, breathing problems, coughing, and wheezing.

Table 7.4, the "Air Quality Forecast and Action Guide," will help you to understand the most suitable environmental conditions for exercise. This guide uses colors to help you distinguish the safest environmental situations. It is dangerous for people with a history of heart disease to exercise outside when the air quality forecast is in the red or orange zone.

### Humidity

The ideal humidity for outdoor exercise is less than 45 percent. With an increase in humidity, the air becomes saturated with its own moisture. This becomes a problem when the temperature and humidity are both high. As the body temperature increases, the blood vessels in and near the skin surface widen to allow the blood to lose its warmth by sweating. But if the air is saturated with its own moisture, this evaporation cannot occur; this may result in a dangerous increase in your body temperature. With high humidity levels, you may want to exercise indoors, or try doing what others do to escape summer humidity—go to the mountains or ocean!

### Wind Velocity

The ideal wind velocity for outdoor exercise is less than 15 mph. During cold-weather months, wind can make the temperature feel much colder. During the summer months, a slight breeze is considered favorable to help prevent stagnant air and improve the air quality.

## Altitude

The effects of high altitude on the body vary from person to person. The reduced oxygen available at higher elevations (above 5,000 feet) can affect your exercise performance and can lead to illness if you are not adequately acclimated. Consult your doctor before setting out for a high-altitude region. High altitudes could cause an increase in angina. You should know these common physical responses associated with poor acclimation:

- increased fatigue
- slight dizziness
- mild shortness of breath
- vague feeling of uneasiness
- mild palpitations or rapid heart rate
- headaches
- restless sleep
- thirst

Don't panic. You can minimize these effects by taking the first three days at higher elevation slow and easy. When you first arrive, cut back on your exercise program by about 50 percent, then slowly increase your level as you tolerate it comfortably over about one week. Factors like overeating and heavy salt intake can intensify high-altitude effects. The effects of alcohol can be exaggerated, so excessive alcohol consumption can be dangerous. Dehydration is more common in higher altitudes, too, so you should increase fluid intake.

Here are some symptoms which are not normal for high altitudes and for which you should seek medical attention:

- new, additional, or unexplained chest pain
- ankle swelling
- alarming shortness of breath
- unusual coughing
- labored breathing

## Varied Terrain

When exercising in areas of varied terrain, hills, or uneven surfaces, reduce your exercise intensity. Walking or biking up a hill

**TABLE 7.4**   Air Quality Forecast and Action Guide

| AIR QUALITY | WEATHER CONDITIONS | ENVIRONMENTAL ACTION |
|---|---|---|
| **UNHEALTHFUL** (CODE RED) | Hot (mid-90s to 100s), hazy, and humid. | **WHEN THE AIR QUALITY REACHES UNHEALTHFUL LEVELS:** |
| | Stagnant air, little or no wind. | Children and elderly individuals should reduce outdoor activities. |
| | Little chance of rain. | Healthy individuals should limit strenuous outdoor work or exercise. |
| | Stationary high-pressure system with sunny skies. | Individuals with heart or respiratory ailments, emphysema, asthma, or chronic bronchitis should limit their outdoor activities. |
| | | If breathing becomes difficult, move indoors. |
| | | **WHEN AIR QUALITY IS FORECAST TO REACH UNHEALTHFUL LEVELS, RESIDENTS ARE STRONGLY URGED TO:** |

## APPROACHING UNHEALTHFUL (CODE ORANGE)

Temperatures in the upper 80s to low 90s.

Light winds.

Slow-moving high-pressure system with sunny skies.

Limit driving and, when possible, combine errands.

Use area bus and rail lines, or share a ride to work.

Avoid mowing lawns with gasoline-powered mowers.

Refuel cars after dusk.

## WHEN AIR QUALITY APPROACHES UNHEALTHFUL LEVELS, RESIDENTS ARE URGED TO:

Refuel cars after dusk to limit daytime pollution releases.

Avoid mowing lawns with gasoline-powered mowers.

Share a ride or drive only their newest, best-maintained vehicle.

continued on next page

**TABLE 7.4** *continued*

| AIR QUALITY | WEATHER CONDITIONS | ENVIRONMENTAL ACTION |
|---|---|---|
| **MODERATE** (CODE YELLOW) | Mild summer temperatures (upper 70s to mid-80s). | **WHEN AIR QUALITY IS IN THE MODERATE RANGE, RESIDENTS SHOULD:** |
| | Light to moderate winds (15 knots or less). | Consolidate trips and errands. |
| | High-pressure system with partly cloudy or sunny skies. | Limit idling when possible. |
| **GOOD** (CODE GREEN) | Cool summer temperatures (mid-70s to low 80s). | **THROUGHOUT THE OZONE SMOG SEASON (MAY THROUGH SEPTEMBER), RESIDENTS SHOULD MAKE AN EXTRA EFFORT TO:** |
| | Windy conditions (15–20 knots or higher). | carpool, use transit, bike, or walk when possible. |
| | Heavy or steady rain. | Keep cars and boats tuned up. |
| | Passing cold front carries pollution out of area. | Use environmentally safe paints and cleaning products. |

# INTERPRETING AIR QUALITY INDEX READINGS:

Each metropolitan area calculates an Air Quality Index (AQI) reading. Listen for this number from your meteorologist and decide whether the air quality is safe.

| AIR QUALITY INDEX READING (AQI) | CORRESPONDING COLOR-CODED FORECAST |
|---|---|
| 0–50 | Code Green |
| 51–58 | Code Yellow |
| 89–99 | Code Orange |
| 100+ | Code Red |

*Source: The Metropolitan Washington Council of Governments.*

increases the intensity of exercise and your heart rate. Slow your pace as you go up an incline so that you always feel comfortable. Exercising on uneven surfaces increases the risk of strains or sprains. Be careful. Invest in well-designed exercise shoes so that you can spend less time nursing a sprain and more time enjoying exercising on a variety of terrains.

## STRIKING THE RIGHT BALANCE:
### SAFETY AND ADVENTURE

- *Temperature.* Extreme temperatures can influence your ability to exercise comfortably outdoors. Learn what you should and should not do to ensure safety.
- *Air quality.* Poor air quality may cause angina, breathing problems, coughing, and wheezing. Use the "Air Quality Forecast and Action Guide" to help you understand safe and healthful weather conditions for exercise. Codes green and yellow are the best air quality conditions for outdoor exercise for people with heart disease.
- *Altitude.* The reduced oxygen available at higher elevations (above 5,000 feet) can affect your exercise performance and can lead to illness if you are not adequately acclimated. Consult your doctor about traveling to high altitudes and learn the physical responses associated with poor acclimation.
- *Varied terrain.* When walking in areas of varied terrain, hills, or uneven surfaces, reduce your exercise intensity. Exercising on uneven surfaces increases your risk of strains or sprains occurring; be careful.

Regardless of the terrain, climate, air quality, or altitude, it is extremely important that you replace fluids lost during exercise at regular intervals. Water allows the body to function normally by converting the food we eat into energy that we use. Water is lost from the body through breathing, perspiration, and other bodily processes. Weather variations and participation in regular exercise programs should prompt you to replace fluids before the body becomes dehydrated.

### Guidelines for Replacing Fluids

1. Water is the best fluid to drink. Cool water is absorbed more quickly in the body than very cold water. Drinks containing sugar take longer for the body to assimilate and should not serve as a substitute for water. The more sugar in the drink, the longer it will take to absorb.

2. Drink approximately 1 cup of water every fifteen to thirty minutes while exercising. It is also beneficial to drink water before and after exercise.

3. Do not wait until you feel thirsty before you replace fluids. Your body can lose several pounds of water before you feel thirsty.

4. Do not take salt tablets. Sodium lost through perspiration can be easily replaced during your next meal.

5. Early signs of dehydration are anxiety, irritability, and fatigue. If any of these symptoms occur, be sure to stop exercising, find a cool place, and drink several glasses of water.

6. More serious signs of dehydration are dizziness, altered level of consciousness, and an uncoordinated walk. If you have any of these symptoms, seek medical assistance immediately.

7. Adults should drink approximately six to eight glasses of water per day with no regular exercise program. If you participate in regular exercise, increase to more than eight glasses of water on your exercise days.

8. Coffee, tea, and alcohol should not be used as replacement fluids. These beverages cause your body to lose fluid.
9. If you are taking diuretic medicines (medicines causing fluid loss) it is important that water be replaced, because you are even more susceptible to dehydration.

In addition to these important fluid replacement practices, you should try to dress for exercise in a way that will let your body get rid of excess heat. This can reduce the likelihood of injury during exercise.

### *Clothing Considerations for Exercising*

When choosing clothes, feeling good is more important than looking good. As a general practice, don't wear rubberized or plastic-type nonporous clothing; it promotes excessive water loss and reduces the body's ability to safely regulate temperature. If your body is not able to cool itself normally (through sweating), your temperature can rise to extremely dangerous levels.

What you choose to wear on your feet is important, too. Today's exercise shoes are designed for specific activities, with the goals of improving exercise performance and preventing injury. Before buying a pair of shoes, consider the surface on which you will be exercising as well as the type of activity you will be doing. You will want a shoe that has good support and shock-absorbing qualities. The maintenance of your exercise shoes is also important. Shoes with excessive wear and tear place you at greater risk for injury. Check your shoes from time to time, and replace them at intervals of six months to a year depending on how active you are.

Balancing safety and adventure begins with understanding how temperature variations, air quality, altitude, and varied terrain can influence how comfortably and safely you exercise. Following these practices may improve your exercise tolerance outdoors and limit the times you feel distressed. But even when you take these precautions, an injury still may occur during exercise. If this happens, try to remember the mnemonic R-I-C-E (see Table 7.5). It is a practical

**TABLE 7.5    If an Injury Occurs: Remember the Mnemonic R-I-C-E**

| | |
|---|---|
| R is for REST | Wait until an injured part no longer hurts at rest before resuming exercise. Then start activities slowly. |
| I is for ICE | Ice reduces swelling, bleeding, and pain. Apply wrapped ice periodically over the injury for 48 hours. Apply ice no longer than 15 minutes per hour. |
| C is for COMPRESSION | Compression reduces swelling and bleeding. Apply pressure to the injured area using an elastic bandage or other soft cloth. |
| E is for ELEVATION | Elevation reduces swelling and pain. Elevate your leg on a chair or raise your arm over your head periodically. |

first aid approach to treating almost any injury, including those that may occur during exercise.

Every injury is unique. However, as a general rule you should see a doctor in the following situations:

- If you hear a pop or snap with the injury.
- If you lose function of the injured extremity.
- If you have severe pain, or pain that persists for more than two weeks.
- If you injure a joint. Any injured joint should be immobilized until it can be examined by a doctor.
- If you have signs of infection—pus, red streaks, swelling, and/or fever.

## A WIN-WIN SITUATION

Achieving balance depends on commitment. Develop an understanding of your own limitations. With a few adjustments, this knowledge will help you to participate safely in your lifestyle of choice. Participate in your progress, take advantage of educational resources that will help you to understand heart disease better, use medications wisely, and take precautions to ensure safety during exercise at all times.

Lifestyle restrictions related to living with heart disease are guided by easy-to-learn principles. Making these adjustments, whether it is to ensure safety during exercise, travel, or the normal activities of daily living, will help you regain a certain level of confidence and control of your life.

§

## CHAPTER EIGHT

# BACK IN CONTROL AGAIN

A HEALTHY HEART AND A HEALTHY BODY ARE A MATTER OF PERSONAL choice. By reading this book you have learned to accept some responsibility for what happened, understand what lifestyle behaviors you need to change, and make a commitment to do so. A diagnosis of heart disease does not have to be an end. Consider this a new beginning. The sooner you start, the sooner you will reap the rewards.

## SETTING GOALS

The heart is an amazing pump. It moves about 2,100 gallons of blood a day; one million barrels of blood in a lifetime. In one year the heart beats about three million times; in the average seventy-year-old it has beaten more than 2.5 billion times. The heart is strong, and can compensate when it is injured. It can rebound from being mended and repaired to functioning at almost optimal capacity—that is, if you do your part.

Look back at your attitudes before all of this happened. Did you believe that good health would be forever? "It won't happen to me. I'm never sick." Don't fall into the same trap by saying, "It won't happen again." It can. If you stop taking care of yourself, your body is at risk for more problems.

How do you take the information you have learned and begin to make a difference? Goal setting will help you to manage lifestyle changes. These goal-setting strategies will help you be successful.

- Identify the problems. Review chapter 2 and list each risk factor that you need to work on.
- Think big, but start small. Focusing on short-term, achievable goals will give you a feeling of satisfaction and confidence. Long-term goals will give you a focused direction for the future.
- Set goals in concrete terms, such as, "I will walk three days per week for thirty minutes on my lunch hour." Avoid vague goals such as, "I will do my best."
- Avoid setting goals that are broad and complex, or are unrealistic in terms of your ability to accomplish them.
- Share goals with others and seek support for accomplishing them.
- Provide incentives to help yourself succeed. This may motivate you to put forth the effort, persistence, and concentration that is needed.
- Reevaluate your goals on a regular basis and make adjustments in your plan as needed. Goals should always be realistic and achievable.

## STAYING MOTIVATED

What are the secrets to success? Why do some people find it easy to stay committed and others just throw up their hands and say, "I can't do it!" We asked individuals participating in cardiac rehabilitation programs ranging in time from six months to thirteen years. Overall, they felt that one must recognize that recovery is a process, not an end point. You won't wake up one day and say, "I'm recovered!" Learn to accept small steps forward, and occasional slips backward. Always keep focused on the long-term goals of preserving your health and quality of life. Make changes because you want to do it, not because your doctor or spouse is forcing you.

On a day-to-day basis, you can help yourself stay motivated by following some of the suggestions that have worked for these successful individuals:

- Leave motivational messages to yourself on the refrigerator.
- Schedule an appointment to exercise on your daily calendar.
- Keep a graph of your weekly weight next to the scale.
- Find a role model and follow his/her example.
- Join a cardiac rehabilitation program in your community.
- Keep a record of your progress regarding risk factors that trouble you.
- Announce to family and friends that you are committed to healthy living.
- Educate yourself. Learn what the outcomes will be if you don't take care of yourself.
- Join a support group.
- Find a substitute activity that you enjoy for something you are giving up.
- Encourage yourself—tell yourself you can do it.
- Learn from past setbacks. What was it that triggered the setback, and how can you keep it from happening again.

The greatest motivation will come from seeing the results of the changes you make. You will feel and look better, and your outlook for the future will improve.

## DEALING WITH SETBACKS

Setbacks can come in a number of different ways. You can have a complication related to your health which requires further medical evaluation and treatment. You can have an emotional setback related to letting yourself become overwhelmed with fear, anxiety, or depression. Or, you can have a setback related to managing your risk factors. You may feel that even though you are doing everything within your control, a particular problem such as cholesterol or weight is not improving as you'd hoped. Remember, no matter how well you are progressing toward a goal, you will still hit roadblocks along the way. Managing heart disease is no different than progress toward any other goal in your life. Setbacks are to be expected. What is important is how you view and manage setbacks.

Bill has been participating in a cardiac rehabilitation program for the past seven years. He works hard at managing his heart disease with varying degrees of success. He exercises regularly, but diet and stress management continue to be a challenge. He doesn't view setbacks as defeats, but rather as problems. "I don't have setbacks—just problems. Everyone has problems, even if you don't have heart disease. So when a problem comes up with my health, I just deal with it—just like I would any other problem in my life."

Bill is confident that he can overcome his problems. If you have confidence that you have the skills to meet new challenges, you will rise to meet them. If you lack confidence in your abilities, you may feel powerless, helpless, hopeless, and unable to take on new tasks. Your energy will be consumed by these negative emotions.

Setbacks can be an opportunity for you to reflect on where you have come from, where you are at, and where you would like to go from here. It is a time for reevaluation. What has been working for you? What needs to be adjusted? What resources could you use that you have not tapped into before? What can you learn from this setback that will prevent it from happening again?

During times like this, it is important to keep in mind that you are in control. During this period of reevaluation, question all the factors that could impact your recovery. Are you satisfied with your relationship with your doctor? Are you getting the support you need to aid you in your recovery? Should you consider private counseling, individual nutrition counseling, a cardiac rehabilitation program, or a cardiac support group?

Explore your own creative alternatives to managing your heart disease. To some extent, many of your health behaviors have been dictated by doctors or other members of your health care team. What strategies can you come up with that will make the changes a more natural progression? Perhaps taking a heart-healthy cooking class, or exploring yoga or meditation as a stress management tool would be a more appealing alternative. Strategies that you select yourself to help manage your risk factors will be more likely to lead to success.

### A NOTE TO FAMILY AND FRIENDS

Everyone is different when it comes to adapting to change. We all have different attitudes, beliefs, skills, and knowledge that can either help or hinder our progress in this area. Some people adapt to change naturally, while others find it much more challenging. Despite the individual nature of change, the process is the same for everyone. One model of behavioral change developed by James Prochaska and Carlo DiClemente helped us to learn that making behavioral changes occurs in several stages. They found that people move back and forth (in no specific order) from each stage to another until finally they reach a point of success—sustaining their desired behavior for a long time. Here are the stages that they talked about and some tips for what you can do to provide support every step of the way:

*continued*

**A NOTE** *continued*

**PRECONTEMPLATION:** A period of resistance. No intention of changing an undesirable health behavior in the next six months.

- Encourage person to practice healthy habits.
- Provide information to help the person understand healthy lifestyle behaviors.

**CONTEMPLATION:** Beginning to think about making changes in the next six months. Recognize a problem exists and have been motivated to change.

- Encourage activities that increase awareness of the problem behavior, its impact on health and quality of life, how to change the behavior, and the benefits of changing. Use this book as your guide.
- Give supportive feedback to help the person feel confident that he or she can succeed in changing unhealthy habits.

**PREPARATION:** Planning to change in the next month.

- Help the person to "get ready" by encouraging commitment.
- Remind the person that changes do not need to be made all at once; he or she should think big but start small.

**ACTION:** Making a change (one day to six months).

- Provide rewards when the person successfully avoids his or her unhealthy behaviors.
- Assist in removing objects in the person's environment that trigger the problem behavior.

- Try to get the person to talk to you about why he or she is reverting to old, bad habits.
- Help the person to see his or her new behavior as a positive change.

**MAINTENANCE:** Able to continue process for over six months.

- Congratulate the person for their success.
- Remind the person to avoid cues that might trigger a relapse.
- Remind the person of current success in changing.

*Source: "The Role of Social Support in the Modification of Risk Factors for Cardiovascular Disease," in,* Social Support and Cardiovascular Disease *by T. L. Amick and J. K. Ockene. S. A. Shumaker and S. M. Czajkowski, eds. New York: Plenum Press, 1994 (p.266). Copyright 1994 by Plenum Press. Adapted with permission.*

## THE POWER OF PERCEPTION

What is the impact of being diagnosed with heart disease on your self-esteem, your internal sense of physical and emotional strength? During the early stages of recovery, you may struggle with fears about the loss of control of your future, or the ability to work, or the end of independence. As these issues are resolved, you may find that what was initially an assault to your sense of well-being can ultimately have a positive impact on your life.

You may be surprised to hear what individuals like you who have been diagnosed with heart disease and are further down the road to recovery are telling us. Sometimes the best advice comes from those who have been there. Many say this was a wake-up call; it may be the best thing that ever happened to them. Listen to what they are saying:

- "I've learned to prioritize. I can more clearly see what is important in my life."
- "I have a new enthusiasm for simple pleasures. I like to garden, I like to hear a good joke, I like to watch old movies. Before, I wouldn't take time for these things."
- "I have a better relationship with my wife. I have gotten rid of so many things that caused me stress that I can enjoy what is important to me."
- "I'm in the best shape I've ever been in. I'm stronger, I have more endurance, I'm not as tired all the time."
- "I'm eating better than I ever have, and I'm enjoying my food."
- "I am able to deal with work pressures better. I realize what is important and what is not."
- "I lost weight and I look and feel great!"
- "I worked out a long-standing feud with my son. I realize life is a gift. I have to treasure it while I have it."
- "I exercise and eat better. I proved to my girlfriend that I would survive, so she agreed to marry me!"

## A HEALTHY BALANCE, A NEW BEGINNING

In this book you have learned the basics to begin your new life. The key to your success is to maintain a positive outlook. You can recover; you can make the changes you need to make; good will come out of this situation in a variety of ways. If you take charge, you will be stronger physically and emotionally. Our wish is that you have a renewed hope for a happy and healthier future.

§

# RESOURCES

NOTE: Information obtained from these resources is not intended to substitute for advice by your doctor.

## ASSOCIATIONS AND ORGANIZATIONS

American Association for Cardiovascular
and Pulmonary Rehabilitation
7611 Elmwood Avenue, Suite 201
Middletown, WI 53526
(608) 831-6989

- Provides directory of cardiac rehabilitation programs in the United States

American Diabetes Association
1660 Duke Street
Alexandria, VA 22314
1-800-232-3472

- Publication, *Healthy Living*
- Information for individuals with diabetes
- Patient information representative available

American Dietetic Association
216 West Jackson Boulevard, Suite 800
Chicago, IL 60606-6995
(312) 899-0040
Consumer Nutrition Hotline
1-800-366-1655

- Provides dietitian referrals in your area
- Specific dietary questions can be answered by calling:
  (900) CALL-AN-RD or (900) 225-5267 (fee for service)
- Recorded messages are available on current news and topics
  such as successful weight loss strategies and debunking myths
- Provides specific messages to certain cities (for example,
  recalls and health warnings)
- Web page: http://www.eatright.org/publications.html

American Heart Association
7270 Greenville Avenue
Dallas, TX 75231
1-800-242-8721

- Provides information on heart disease and stroke
- News releases

American Lung Association
1726 M Street, NW
Washington, DC 20036
(202) 785-3355

- Educational pamphlets are available: asthma, tuberculosis,
  asbestos, and smoking cessation
- Environmental health publications
- Tobacco legislation information and news

Citizens for Public Action on Blood Pressure and Cholesterol
P.O. Box 30374
Bethesda, MD 20824
(301) 770-1711

- Distributes educational materials on blood pressure
  and cholesterol control

Cooper Institute for Aerobics Research
12330 Preston Road
Dallas, TX 75230
1-800-444-5764

- "Health-Fitness Information Line" answers your health-related questions
- Web page: http://www.cooperinst.org

Heartline
9500 Euclid Avenue
Mail Code EE37
Cleveland, OH 44195
(216) 444-3690

- Newsletter subscription available

Heartmates, Inc.
1-800-946-3331

- Information for spouses and families living with heart disease

Medic Alert Identification
Medic Alert Foundation
Turlock, CA 95381-1009
1-800-ID-ALERT

- Access to medical identification information

Mended Hearts, Inc.
7272 Greenville Avenue
Dallas, TX 75231
(214) 706-1442

- Support group for individuals with heart disease
- Members receive a quarterly publication
- Contact Mended Hearts, Inc. to find a local chapter near you

## GOVERNMENT RESOURCES

National Cholesterol Education Program
National Institutes of Health
7200 Wisconsin Avenue
Bethesda, MD 20824
(301) 251-1222

- All resources are listed on Web page:
  http://www.nhlbi.nih.gov/nhlbi/nhlbi.htm

National Diabetes Information Clearinghouse
One Information Way
Bethesda, MD 20892-3560

- Publications on diabetes are available to consumers
- Resources are listed on Web page: http://www.niddk.nih.gov

National Health Information Center (NHIC)
P.O. Box 1133
Washington, DC 20013-1133
1-800-336-4797

- The Department of Health & Human Services (Office of Disease Prevention and Health Promotion) provides a health information referral service; this service specializes in putting people with health and medical questions in contact with public and private organizations
- Write for a list of toll-free numbers for health information

National Heart, Lung, & Blood Institute
P.O. Box 30105
Bethesda, MD 20824-0105
(301) 251-1222

- All resources are listed on Web page:
  http://www.nhlbi.nih.gov/nhlbi/nhlbi.htm

National Library of Medicine
1-800-272-4787

- Provides information and assistance on MEDLINE and other databases. You may search databases to locate current abstracts of articles on a variety of topics related to heart disease; approximately 30,000 new citations appear each month on MEDLINE
- Assistance is provided with citations and reference information on a subject
- Interlibrary loans are available
- Resources are listed on Web page: http://www.nlm.nih.gov

U.S. Government Printing Office
Consumer Information Center
Department 420W
Pueblo, CO 81009

- Resources are listed on Web page: http://www.pueblo.gsa.gov/food.htm

## AREA HOSPITALS

Many hospitals offer special health education programs for people in their communities. Contact hospitals nearest you for more information.

## LIBRARY RESOURCES

*The AT&T Toll-Free National 800 Directory:*
- A reference to access toll-free numbers for health information.

*Consumer Health Information Source Book:*
- A reference of information clearinghouses, useful books, and other resources.

*Health Information Directory:*
- A reference of organizations, publications, libraries, and health services.

*Self-Help Source Book:*
- A reference of over 700 organizations that can help you find a support group.

## BOOKS

Anderson, Jean, and Barbara Deskins. *The Nutrition Bible.* New York: Quill/William Morrow, 1995.
(General nutrition reference)

Carlson, Karen J., M.D., Stephanie A. Eisenstat, M.D., and Terra Zigoryn. *The Harvard Guide to Women's Health.* Cambridge, Mass.: Harvard University Press, 1996.
(Provides specific references for women)

Clayman, Charles B., M.D., ed. *American Medical Association Encyclopedia of Medicine.* New York: Random House, 1989.
(Overview of specific medical conditions)

Connolly, J. *How to Find the Best Doctors, Hospitals, and HMOs.* New York: Castle Connolly Medical Ltd., 1995.

Ferguson, Tom. *Health On-Line.* Reading, Mass.: Addison-Wesley Publishing Company, 1996.
(How to find health information and support groups in cyberspace)

Glanze, Walter D., Kenneth N. Anderson, and Lois E. Anderson, eds. *The Mosby Medical Encyclopedia.* New York: Signet, 1992.
(Medical dictionary)

Guthrie, Diana, and Richard Guthrie, M.D. *The Diabetes Sourcebook*, 3d ed. Los Angeles: Lowell House, 1997.

Kelley, David B., et al., eds., *American Diabetes Association Complete Guide to Diabetes.* Alexandria, Va.: American Diabetes Association, 1996.

Netzer, Corinne T. *The Encyclopedia of Food Values.* New York: Dell, 1992.
(Diet planning and general food facts)

U.S. Pharmacopedia. *Complete Drug Reference.* Consumer Reports Books, A Division of Consumers Union, Yonkers, N.Y.: 1996.
(Understanding your prescription medicines)

———. *The Guide to Heart Medications.* New York: Avon Books, 1996.
(Understanding your prescription medicines)

Wright, J. *The Best Hospitals in America.* Detroit, Mich.: Gale Research, 1995.
(A listing of the top hospitals)

Zaret, Barry L. *The Yale University School of Medicine—Patient's Guide to Medical Tests.* Boston: Houghton Mifflin Company, 1997.

## NEWSLETTERS

Consumer Reports on Health
P.O. Box 52148
Boulder, CO 80321-2148

Mayo Clinic Healthletter
P.O. Box 53889
Boulder, CO 80322-3889

Coronary Club Hotline Letter
(216) 444-3690

Nutrition Action Health Letter
(202) 332-9110

The Harvard Health Letter
(617) 432-1485

The University of California at
Berkeley Wellness Letter
(904) 445-6414

The Johns Hopkins Medical
Letter Health After 50
(904) 446-4675

Women's Health Watch
1-800-829-5921

## COMPUTER LINKS TO HEALTH INFORMATION

American Cancer Society
http://www.cancer.org

- Cancer information, programs, research progress, events, and news
- Tobacco information

American Heart Association (AHA)
http://www.amhrt.org

- Today's News
- What's Your Risk for Heart Disease?
- Heart and Stroke A–Z Guide
- News releases (current and local)
- Home, Health, and Family
- Your Local AHA

Arthritis Foundation
http://www.arthritis.org

- Arthritis Today
- News, facts, and resources

Centers for Disease Control and Prevention
http://www.cdc.gov

- Current news and publications
- Health information, Travelers' Health
- What's New?

Dietary Guidelines
http://www.nalusda.gov/fnic/dga/dga95.html

- Dietary guidelines for Americans
- Information on alcohol, salt, sugar, grains, and fat intake
- Importance of variety in diet

Harvard Medical School
http://www.med.harvard.edu

- Library access
- Electronic journals and publications

Hospitals on the Web
http://neuro-www.mgh.harvard.edu/hospitalweb.nclk

- The Hospital Patient: A Guide for Family and Friends
- Information access to hospitals around the world (growing globally)

International Food Information Council
http://ificinfo.health.org

- Food safety and nutrition information
- Publications
- What's New?

Medical Matrix
http://www.medmatrix.org

- MEDLINE access, journals
- Patient education
- News
- R$_X$ Assist

National Aging Information Center (NAIC)
http://pr.aoa.dhhs.gov/naic/

- Learn about what NAIC can do for you
- Database, eldercare locator
- Calendar of coming events in aging
- Publications

National Health Information Center (NHIC)
http://nhic-nt.health.org

- Health information for consumers from a database of over 1,000 organizations and government offices

National Institutes of Health (NIH)
http://www.nih.gov

- News, events, and health information
- Guide to diseases and conditions under investigation by NIH
- Resource links to consumer health publications

National Institute of Mental Health
http://www.nimh.nih.gov

- Public information on specific mental disorders, diagnoses, and treatment
- News and events

National Library of Medicine
http://www.nlm.nih.gov

- Hot topics, news, special information programs
- Health information, MEDLINE access (free), subscriptions to mailing list, publications, databases, and electronic information services

National Women's Health Information Center
http://www.4woman.org

- Women's health information

Pharmaceutical Information Network
http://www.pharminfo.com

- Drug information
- Effects of common foods on popular drugs
- News and articles
- Cardiovascular, diabetes, cancer, and obesity disease centers
- Cardiology and diabetes discussion groups

Toll-Free Numbers for Health Information *and*
Health Information Resources in the Federal Government,
Sixth Edition
http://odphp.osophs.dhhs.gov/gopher.htm

U.S. Government
HealthFinder™
http://www.healthfinder.gov

- Consumer health information service linking over 600 federal agencies, academic and professional organizations, and non-commercial organizations to provide reliable public information
- Links to state and local health departments
- Links to medical, university, and public libraries
- Links to hotlines, discussion groups, and support groups
- Tour—heart disease and stroke

§

# CURRENT TOPICS IN HEART DISEASE

HEART DISEASE IS A COMPLEX TOPIC. WE KNOW A LOT ABOUT IT, but there is also a great deal more to learn. As research continues, studies present findings about previously unknown factors that may contribute to the prevention, diagnosis, and treatment of heart disease. Scientific research is a long and complex process. As ideas become apparent that may assist in the treatment of heart disease, they require more detailed and widespread validation. Many new theories related to the treatment of heart disease have been appearing in the scientific literature and the general media over the last decade. Although research is not conclusive, there is enough evidence pointing in a specific direction to allow the medical community to establish opinions. The following is a brief summary of some of these topics.

## HORMONE REPLACEMENT THERAPY

Research is convincing that hormone replacement therapy for post-menopausal women offers many benefits. The major advantages are reduction in the risk of heart disease and osteoporosis, and lessening in the symptoms of menopause such as hot flashes and vaginal dryness. The detriments are increased risk of breast cancer with long-term use, and increased risk of endometrial cancer. Your decision about whether to begin or continue to use hormone replacement therapy involves evaluating your risks for heart disease, osteoporosis, breast cancer, and endometrial cancer.

If you are at high risk for heart disease or already have it, then hormone replacement therapy may be a good choice for you. Hormone replacement therapy increases HDL cholesterol (the good cholesterol) and decreases LDL cholesterol (the bad cholesterol). It is also thought that hormone replacement decreases the blood clotting that may cause a heart attack, relaxes blood vessels, and improves the body's response to insulin, keeping blood sugar levels within normal limits. Overall, it is estimated that hormone replacement therapy lowers the risk of coronary artery disease by as much as 44 percent.

Evidence also exists that hormones help to prevent osteoporosis, a thinning of bones that results in bone fractures. Hormones typically stop bone loss, and may even cause a small increase in bone density.

The increased risk of breast cancer in women taking hormone replacement therapy is associated with duration of use, with an increased incidence beginning at five years (1.3 times the average), and increasing to 1.7 times the average after seven years. Evaluating your risk for breast cancer, including family history of breast cancer, will help you and your physician determine the best choice for you.

The increased risk of endometrial cancer (cancer of the uterine lining) for women taking hormone replacement therapy appears to disappear when estrogen and progesterone are taken together. Estrogen alone has been shown to increase the risk of cancer of the uterine lining; however, adding progesterone prevents overgrowth of the endometrium. Therefore, estrogen and progesterone are generally prescribed together for women who have not had a hysterectomy.

Your decision about whether to begin or continue hormone therapy involves evaluating how the various pros and cons affect you. What are your personal risk factors for heart disease, osteoporosis, and breast cancer? You will receive the most benefit from hormone therapy by beginning treatment at menopause and continuing it for the long term. Research continues on this topic with the Women's Health Initiative, a large study looking at the major causes of disease and death in postmenopausal women. In the meantime, your wisest option is to discuss the benefits and risks with your physician in order to come up with the best decision for you based on the current knowledge.

## ALCOHOL

Some areas of research have suggested that daily consumption of moderate amounts of alcohol may reduce your risk of coronary artery disease. Research continues on whether the benefits are from red wine or just alcohol in general. The key is moderate amounts of alcohol daily, which is defined as 5 ounces of wine, 12 ounces of beer, and 1.5 ounces of liquor.

Your doctor will assist you in making decisions about alcohol consumption based on your specific medical history. Excessive alcohol consumption can lead to dependency and can cause heart disease as well as liver disease and strokes, and increases the risk of death caused by accidents. Additionally, alcohol lowers inhibitions and promotes relapse for individuals trying to stop smoking or lose weight.

## ANTIOXIDANTS

Antioxidants include vitamins C and E and beta-carotene. Research suggests that by-products of cell activities over time cause damage to cell walls and may lead to the development of many chronic illnesses associated with aging. Antioxidants may block this action, thereby controlling cell damage and slowing the development and progression of chronic disease.

Numerous factors, including heredity and overall lifestyle, play a role in the development of chronic age-related illness. However, research indicates that antioxidants may also play a significant part in preventing cancer, heart disease, cataracts, and other diseases of the elderly.

Research supports the relationship between intake of vitamin E and vitamin C supplements and a lower incidence of heart disease. Consult your physician about recommended doses. Current ranges include 200–800 IU of vitamin E, and 250–500 mg of vitamin C. Research on beta-carotene has not shown a lower incidence of heart disease, and, in fact, preliminary results showed an increased incidence of lung cancer and lung cancer deaths for individuals taking beta-carotene supplements.

Research continues on the value of antioxidant supplements. Remember that fresh fruits and vegetables are rich in antioxidants. Adults should consume a diet that includes two to four servings of fruit and three to five servings of vegetables daily. Following these dietary guidelines will provide you with the needed amounts of antioxidants.

## HOMOCYSTEINE

In the past few years, research has consistently linked high levels of homocysteine to an increased risk of heart attack. Homocysteine is a type of chemical in the body called an amino acid. High levels of homocysteine in the body are connected to inadequate intake of folate and vitamins $B_6$, and $B_{12}$. When levels of B vitamins are too low in the diet and the blood, homocysteine accumulates and artery-damaging plaque develops, resulting in heart attacks and stroke.

Folate and vitamin $B_6$ are commonly found in leafy green vegetables, fruits, grains, legumes, and fish. Vitamin $B_{12}$ is found in animal products. These findings provide additional support for eating five fruits and vegetables per day which, in addition to providing vitamins, nutrients, electrolytes, and fiber, will also help to control homocysteine levels. Taking vitamin supplements should be done with the advice of your physician. Normal recommendations are to take a daily multivitamin that contains 400 micrograms of folic acid, 2 milligrams of $B_6$, and 1 milligram of $B_{12}$ to be sure you are meeting the RDA for these nutrients.

Research continues on whether routine analysis of homocysteine levels would be a useful screening tool for heart disease prevention. Some studies report that elevated homocysteine levels increase the risk of heart disease by almost three times. Evidence is not clear if homocysteine levels are just an indicator for heart disease, or if bringing homocysteine levels down to normal will decrease the risk for heart disease, as is the case with cholesterol. While the research continues, heed the advice and include five servings of fruits and vegetables in your diet each day.

## CHELATION THERAPY

Chelation therapy is an accepted medical treatment for heavy metal poisoning, including lead poisoning. The theory is that when this chemical comes in contact with a harmful metal, it binds with it and both are excreted from the body. Researchers questioned if this would also bind with the calcium in plaque buildup in the arteries of the heart, and remove the plaque from the body; if so, this could be used as a replacement for heart bypass surgery or angioplasty.

The medical establishment believes that chelation therapy at this point is unproven. One concern is that calcium is being removed from bone in addition to plaque. It is also pointed out that calcium is only a small component of plaque, which also includes scar tissue, cholesterol, fibrin, and other substances. The effect on blood flow of removing calcium in plaque is minimal.

Currently, the greatest flaw in the promotion of chelation therapy is limited valid research on its effectiveness. For this reason, the medical community and organizations such as the American Heart Association have not approved chelation therapy as an acceptable treatment for heart disease.

## ULTRAFAST COMPUTED TOMOGRAPHY

Ultrafast Computed Tomography provides three-dimensional views of the beating heart and flowing blood used to diagnose coronary artery disease. It can be useful in identifying calcium deposits in coronary arteries. A calcium score is calculated; the higher the score, the more likely calcium buildup is present. Further diagnostic testing and treatment is then recommended. The results of using this test as a screening tool for heart disease have been mixed. The presence of calcium deposits in an artery does not necessarily mean an artery is significantly blocked. Additionally, plaque buildup can include scar tissue, cholesterol, fibrin, and other substances, in addition to calcium. For some individuals, the Ultrafast Computed Tomography test would be negative, even though there is plaque buildup present.

## POSITIVE EMISSION TOMOGRAPHY

Positive Emission Tomography is a diagnostic imaging technique which produces three-dimensional images of the heart's blood flow, structure, and cellular metabolism by tracing the release of radioactive substances. Its primary limitation is cost; it is very expensive and therefore less widely used than other diagnostic tools that can provide the same information.

## MAGNETIC RESONANCE IMAGING

Magnetic Resonance Imaging uses radio waves and a powerful magnet to scan the heart. The magnetic pulses generated by the powerful magnet send electromagnetic signals that can be converted into three-dimensional pictures of the heart and coronary arteries. This method has not replaced the coronary angiogram because the pictures are taken of a beating heart and the motion blurs the images, making them difficult to interpret and decreasing the degree of accuracy. Research continues to evaluate the use of MRI for diagnosing heart disease.

§

# SELECTING AN EXERCISE PROGRAM

SELECTING AN EXERCISE PROGRAM THAT IS RIGHT FOR YOU TAKES careful consideration. There is a vast array of options. You can spend under $75 for a good pair of walking shoes and some hand-held weights, or over $5,000 for a state-of-the-art treadmill. Ask yourself these questions:

- What exercise have I done in the past that I enjoyed?
- Do I have any orthopedic limitations that will limit my exercise? (If you have orthopedic problems, such as arthritis or old injuries to bones or joints, consult with your doctor about selecting an exercise program that is best for you.)
- Do I enjoy exercising alone or with the company of friends?
- Where can I find time to fit exercise into my daily routine (days of the week, time of day)?
- If I purchase home exercise equipment, where will it fit in my home?

Answering these questions will help you focus on exercise options that will work for you. Your choices include enrolling in a supervised cardiac rehabilitation center, developing a home exercise program that may include walking or using home exercise equipment, beginning an outdoor walking program, and/or participating in an exercise program at a local health club or recreation center.

## CARDIAC REHABILITATION

If you have recently been diagnosed with heart disease, the best option during the first three months of recovery is a supervised cardiac rehabilitation program. These programs are available at most hospitals (see appendix A). They provide an initial three-month program of supervised exercise that is specifically designed based on your medical history, and guidance and education on risk factor management. Most insurance companies will provide coverage for a portion of the cost of the program.

## HEALTH CLUBS

Selecting a health club takes some careful investigation. The range of contract options and services available can be confusing. Issues to evaluate before selecting a health club include:

### *Proximity to Your Home or Work*
You will not continue a routine of regular exercise at a health club that is not convenient for you. Choose a health club that is within ten minutes of your home or work. Check the hours of operation to be sure it is open when you want to exercise.

### *Contract/Payment Options*
Sifting through the realm of contract types and payment options can be bewildering. Make a list of what you are looking for and

compare it to the options available to find one that meets your needs. Don't fall for health club extras that are above and beyond what your needs or abilities are. You should be prepared to discuss the initiation fee, payment options, and membership types. Ask about the availability of a trial membership.

### Qualifications and Availability of Staff

Individuals who will provide guidance on proper use of exercise equipment and development and progression of your exercise program should have proper training. Ask about the qualifications of staff and check staff availability at the time of day you will exercise.

### Maintenance and Availability of Equipment

Visit the health club at the time of day you will be exercising. Is the equipment you will be using available to you and in good repair? Are there time limits to using the equipment?

## HOME EXERCISE EQUIPMENT

Selecting a home exercise program begins with identifying what type of exercise will work best for you. The goal is an exercise program that you enjoy, that provides you with an aerobic workout, and that does not risk injury to bones, muscles, or joints. Consider the following when selecting home exercise equipment:

1. Never buy equipment without trying it first.
2. Wear your exercise clothes when you are shopping so that you can try the equipment.
3. Look for a retailer with knowledgeable salespeople and a service department.
4. Find out if your equipment comes assembled, if it has a warranty, if it can be traded in or upgraded, and if it can be returned.
5. Know the features you want before you shop. Equipment that

has a modest number of features is less expensive than that with many extras.

6. Examine brand name vs. non-brand name models. Examine equipment for quality, price, noise, safety, convenience, smoothness, and comfort. What are the advantages and disadvantages of each?

7. Be skeptical of products with weight loss claims that are too good to be true.

8. If you have difficulty checking your pulse accurately, consider purchasing a pulse meter (a device that automatically registers your pulse). These are available in most sporting goods stores. The most reliable models consist of a transmitter belt worn around your chest that transmits your pulse to a watch.

The most common types of home exercise equipment are treadmills, stationary bicycles, stair climbers, and cross-country ski machines. Sorting through the maze of different brands, options, and prices when shopping for exercise equipment can be confusing. The following information will help you to ask the right questions and be an informed consumer.

### Treadmills

A treadmill should be easy to use and should be stable when your foot lands. The length of the belt should allow for a normal walking gait as well as jogging. Adjustments for speed and incline should be available. Options packages may also include electronic programming that automatically varies speed and incline.

Nonmotorized treadmills require the individual to control the speed based on the pace of his or her walk. Extra effort is needed to move the belt, and a steady pace is not guaranteed. Motorized treadmills provide settings that set the miles per hour and grade or elevation. Considerations include the length and width of the walking surface (a minimum of 8 feet by 5 feet), and the horsepower of the motor. Drawbacks to motorized treadmills include noise and the possible need for a special electrical outlet to handle power needs.

### Exercise Bikes

Exercise bikes come in a variety of styles including upright, recumbent, and dual-action bikes (handlebars move back and forth while pedaling). All three types should include a selection for monitoring resistance, a measurement of revolutions per minute, and a seat adjustment. The upright bicycle is closest to an outdoor bike. Another alternative is to purchase a bike stand that converts your outdoor bike to a stationary bike. The recumbent bicycle usually provides a more comfortable seat and is a good option for individuals with back or weight problems. The dual-action bicycle is a total body workout that allows you to use your arms and legs simultaneously, propelling handlebars in a forward and backward motion while pedaling.

Selecting the right type of bicycle depends on comfort and consideration of any specific bone, muscle, or joint problems. Look into trial membership specials offered at area health clubs. This can provide you the opportunity to experiment with the different types of bicycles available.

### Stair Climbers

Stair climbers provide aerobic exercise by simulating actual stair climbing, varying the stepping resistance and/or the height of the steps. Options include electronic programming that automatically varies stepping resistance and dual-action steppers that exercise arms and legs. When trying out equipment, look for smoothness in the stepping action and sturdiness of the pedals and handles. Be aware that stair climbing is a high-intensity workout, and careful monitoring of your heart rate response to exercise will be necessary to ensure that you stay in your target heart rate range.

## *Cross-Country Ski Machines*

Cross-country ski machines provide aerobic exercise by simulating cross-country skiing. Your feet glide back and forth and your arms move forward and backward, providing a total body workout. For some individuals it is a favorite exercise, but others find it difficult to master the motion required. Options include independent motion of skis, which requires the individual to propel the skis, or dependent motion, which moves the opposite ski backward automatically when you move one ski forward. Resistance settings and incline should also be adjustable.

§

CHAPTER ONE

Gray, H. *Anatomy of the Human Body.* Philadelphia: Lea and Febiger, 1985.

Hollingshead, W. H. and C. Rosse. *Textbook of Anatomy.* 4th ed. New York: Harper and Row, 1985.

Kirklin, J. W. and B. G. Barrat-Boyes. *Cardiac Surgery.* 2d ed. New York: Churchill Livingstone, 1993.

Tortora, G. J. *Principles of Anatomy and Physiology.* New York: Collins College, 1993.

Willerson, J. T. and J.N. Cohn, eds. *Cardiovascular Medicine.* New York: Churchill Livingstone, 1995.


CHAPTER TWO

Agency for Health Care Policy and Research. "Smoking Cessation Clinical Practice Guidelines." April 1996.

American College of Sports Medicine. *Guidelines for Exercise Testing and Prescription.* 5th ed. Philadelphia: Lea and Febiger, 1995.

Assaf, A. R., R. A. Carleton, T. M. Lasater, and H. A. Feldman. "The Pawtucket Heart Health Program: Community Changes in Cardiovascular Risk Factors and Projected Disease Risk." *American Journal of Public Health* 85: 77–85 (1995).

Bray, G. A. and D. S. Gray. "Obesity." *Western Journal of Medicine* 149: 429 41 (1988).

Connett, J., D. R. Jacobs, A. S. Leon, and R. Rauramaa. "Leisure Time Physical Activity and Risk of Coronary Heart Disease and Death: The Multiple Risk Factor Intervention Trial." *Journal of American Medical Association* 285: 2388–95 (1987).

Connett, J. and A. Leon. "Physical Activity and 10.5 Year Mortality in the Multiple Risk Factor Intervention Trial." *International Journal of Epidemiology* 20: 690–7 (1991).

Framingham Heart Study, Section 37. "The Probability of Developing Certain Cardiovascular Diseases in Eight Years at Specified Values of Some Characteristics." (August 1987).

Friedman, Meyer, M.D. and Ray Rosenman, M.D. *Type A Behavior and Your Heart*. New York: Ballantine Books, 1974.

Manson, J. E., et al. "Body Weight and Mortality among Women." *New England Journal of Medicine* 333:677–685 (1995).

National Cholesterol Education Program, National Heart, Lung, and Blood Institute, National Institute of Health. "Expert Panel on Detection, Evaluation, and Treatment of High Blood Cholesterol in Adults." (1993).

*"Physical Activity and Cardiovascular Health."* NIH Consens Statement. 13(3):1–33 (Dec. 18–20, 1995).

Report of the Joint National Committee on Detection, Evaluation, and Treatment of High Blood Pressure, 1993.

Surgeon General Report on the Health Benefit of Smoking Cessation, 1990.

U.S. Public Health Service. "Healthy People 2000: National Health Promotion and Disease Prevention Objectives—Fall Report with Commentary." Department of Health and Human Services Publication 91-50212. Washington, D.C., 1991.

Williams, Redford B. *Hostility and the Heart in Mind Body Medicine*. D. Goleman and J. Gurin, eds. New York: Consumer Reports Books, 1993.

## CHAPTER THREE

American Heart Association. *Heart at Work*. 1993.

Amick, T. L. and J. K. Ockene. "The Role of Social Support in the Modification of Risk Factors for Cardiovascular Disease." In *Social*

*Support and Cardiovascular Disease.* S. A. Shumaker and S. M. Czajkowski, eds. New York: Plenum Press, 1994.

Bakker, C., M. Bogdonoff, and H. Hellerstein. "Heart Disease and Sex." *Medical Aspects of Human Sexuality* 5: 24 (1971).

Bandura, Albert. *Social Learning Theory.* Englewood Cliffs, N.J.: Prentice-Hall, 1987.

———. "Toward a Unifying Theory of Behavior Change." *Psychological Review* 84: 191–215 (1977).

Brownell, Kelly, G. Alan Marlatt, Edward Lichtenstein, and G. Terence Wilson. "Understanding and Preventing Relapse." *American Psychologist* 41: 765–82 (1986).

Budnick, Herbert. *Heart to Heart.* Santa Fe, N. Mex.: Health Press, 1991.

Cooper, A. J. "Myocardial Infarction and Advice on Sexual Activity." *Practitioner* 229: 575 (1985).

Davidson, D. M., C. B. Taylor, and R. F. DeBusk. "Factors Influencing Return to Work After Myocardial Infarction or Coronary Artery Bypass Surgery." *Cardiac Rehabilitation* 10: 1 (1979).

Dennis, C., N. Houston-Miller, R. G. Schwartz, et al. "Early Return to Work After Uncomplicated Myocardial Infarction: Results of a Randomized Trial." *Journal of American Medical Association* 260: 214 (1988).

Franklin, B. A. "Getting Patients Back to Work After Myocardial Infarction or Coronary Artery Bypass Surgery." *Physician and Sports Medicine* 14: 183 (1986).

Kenney, W. Larry, R. Humphrey, and C. X. Bryant, eds. *Guidelines for Exercise Testing and Prescription.* 5th ed. Baltimore, Md.: Williams & Wilkins, 1995.

Larson, J. L., M. W. McNaughton, J. W. Kennedy, et al. "Heart Rate and Blood Pressure Responses to Sexual Activity and a Stair-Climbing Test." *Heart and Lung* 9: 1025 (1980).

Levin, Rhoda. *Heartmates.* Englewood Cliffs, N.J.: Prentice Hall, 1987.

Levine, S. B. "Marital Sexual Dysfunction: Introductory Concepts." *Annals of Internal Medicine* 84: 1133 (1976).

Miller, N. H., D. Gossard, and C. B. Taylor. "Advice to Resume Sexual Activity After Myocardial Infarction." *Circulation* 70 II–134: (1984).

Papadopoulos, C. "Coronary Artery Disease and Sexuality." In *Sexual Aspects of Cardiovascular Disease.* New York: Praeger, 1989.

———. "Sexual Problems/Interventions." *Rehabilitation of the Coronary Patient.* 3d ed. Nanette Wenger and Herman Hellerstein, eds. New York: Churchill Livingstone, 1992.

Pollin, Irene and Susan Golant. *Taking Charge: How to Master the Eight Most Common Fears of Long-Term Illness.* New York: Random House, 1994.

Raft, D., D. C. McKee, K. A. Popio, et al: "Life Adaptation After Percutaneous Transluminal Coronary Angioplasty and Coronary Artery Bypass Grafting." *American Journal of Cardiology* 56: 395 (1985).

Smith, Hugh. "Return to Work." *Rehabilitation of the Coronary Patient.* 3d ed. Nanette Wenger and Herman Hellerstein, eds. New York: Churchill Livingstone, 1992.

Sotile, Wayne M. *Psychosocial Interventions for Cardiopulmonary Patients.* Champaign, Ill.: Human Kinetics, 1996.

Wallston, Barbara, Sheryle Alagna, Brenda McEvoy DeVellis, and Robert DeVellis. "Social Support and Physical Health." *Health Psychology,* 2: 367–91 (1983).

## CHAPTER FOUR

Allen, T. E., R. J. Byrd, and D. P. Smith. "Hemodynamic Consequences of Circuit Weight Training." *Research Quarterly in Exercise and Sport* 47: 299–306 (1976).

The American Association of Cardiovascular and Pulmonary Rehabilitation. *Guidelines for Cardiac Rehabilitation Programs.* Champaign, Ill.: Human Kinetics, 1995.

Berlin, J. A. and G. A. Colditz. "A Meta Analysis of Physical Activity in the Prevention of Coronary Heart Disease." *American Journal of Epidemiology* 132: 612–28 (1990).

Blair, S. and M. Morrow. "Surgeon General's Report on Physical Fitness." *American College of Sports Medicine's Health & Fitness Journal* 1: 14–17 (1997).

Borg, G. V. "Psychophysical Basis of Perceived Exertion." *Medicine and Science in Sports and Exercise* 14: 377–81 (1982).

Chandrasheckhar, Y. and I. S. Anand. "Exercise As a Coronary Protective Factor." *American Heart Journal* 122: 1723–39 (1991).

Dishman, R. K., ed. *Exercise Adherence: Its Impact on Public Health.* Champaign, Ill.: Human Kinetics, 1988.

Fletcher, G. F., V. F. Froelicher, L. H. Hartley, et al. "Exercise Standards: A Statement for Health Professionals from the American Heart Association." *Circulation* 82: 2286–322 (1990).

Frankin, B. A., S. Gordon, and G. C. Timmis. "Amount of Exercise Necessary for the Patient with Coronary Heart Disease." *American Journal of Cardiology* 69: 1426–31 (1992).

Hillgass, E. A. and H. S. Sadowsky, eds. *Essentials of Cardiopulmonary Physical Therapy.* Philadelphia: W.B. Saunders, 1994.

Kenney, W. Larry, R. Humphrey, and C. X. Bryant, eds. *Guidelines for Exercise Testing and Prescription.* 5th ed. Baltimore, Md.: Williams & Wilkins, 1995.

Leon, A. S., C. Certo, P. Cosmoss, et al. "Position Paper of the American Association of Cardiovascular and Pulmonary Rehabilitation: Scientific Evidence of the Value of Cardiac Rehabilitation Services with Emphasis on Patients with Myocardial Infarction—Section I: Exercise Conditioning Component." *Journal of Cardiopulmonary Rehabilitation* 10: 79–87 (1990).

McArdle, William, Frank Katch, and Victor Katch. *Exercise Physiology, Energy, Nutrition, and Human Performance.* 4th ed. Baltimore, Md.: Williams & Wilkins, 1996.

Morris, C. K. and V. F. Froelicher. "Cardiovascular Benefits of Improved Exercise Capacity. *Sports Medicine* 16: 225–36 (1993).

Noble, B. J. "Clinical Applications of Perceived Exertion." *Medicine and Science in Sports and Exercise* 14: 406–411 (1982).

*"Physical Activity and Cardiovascular Health."* NIH Consens Statement, 13(3): 1–33 (Dec. 18–20, 1995).

Pollack, M. L. and D. H. Schmidt. *Heart Disease and Rehabilitation.* 3d ed. Champaign, Ill.: Human Kinetics, 1995.

U.S. Department of Health and Human Services. "Healthy People 2000: National Health Promotion & Disease Prevention Objectives." Public Health Service, 1991.

Verrill, D., E. Shoup, G. McElveen, et al. "Resistive Exercise Training in Cardiac Patients." *Sports Medicine* 13: 171–93 (1996).

Williams, M. *Exercise Testing and Training in the Elderly Cardiac Patient.* Champaign, Ill.: Human Kinetics, 1995.


CHAPTER FIVE

Mahan, L. K. and S. Escott-Stump. *Food, Nutrition, and Diet Therapy.* 9th ed. Philadelphia: W. B. Saunders Co., 1996.

National Research Council. "Recommended Dietary Allowances." Washington, D.C.: National Academy Press, 1989.

Shils, M. E., J. A. Olson, and M. Shike. *Modern Nutrition in Health and Disease*. Philadelphia: Lea and Febiger, 1994.

U.S. Department of Agriculture. "The Food Guide Pyramid." Home and Garden Bulletin no. 252, Human Nutritional Information Service, Washington, D.C. (1992).

U.S. Department of Agriculture and U.S. Department of Health and Human Services. "Nutrition and Your Health: Dietary Guidelines for Americans." Home and Garden Bulletin no. 232, Government Printing Office (1990).

## CHAPTER SIX

Aiken, L. H. and T. F. Henricks. "Systematic Relaxation As a Nursing Intervention Technique with Open Heart Surgery Patients." *Nursing Research* 20, no. 3: 212–16 (1971).

Albrecht. *Stress and the Manager: Making It Work for You*. Englewood Cliffs, N.J.: Prentice-Hall, Inc., 1979.

Allen, R. J. *Human Stress: Its Nature and Control*. Minnesota: Burgess Press, 1983.

Anthony, J. and J. Hurley. "Humor Therapy: To Heal Is to Make Happy." *Nursing Clinical Currents* 2, no. 1: 1–4 (1989).

Bandura, Albert. *Social Learning Theory*. New Jersey: Prentice-Hall, Inc., 1987.

———. "Toward a Unifying Theory of Behavior Change." *Psychological Review* 84: 191–215 (1977).

Beck, A. T. "Cognitive Approaches to Stress Management." In *Principles and Practice of Stress Management*. R. L. Woolfolk and P. M. Lehrer, eds. New York: Guilford Press, 1984.

Bennett, Robert, Kurt Hanks, and Gerrold Palsipher. *Gaining Control*. Salt Lake City, Utah: Franklin International Institute, Inc., 1987.

Benson, Herbert, and M. Kippler. *The Relaxation Response*. New York: Avon, 1976.

Benson, Herbert, and Eileen Stuart. *The Wellness Workbook: A Comprehensive Guide to Maintaining Health and Treating Stress-Related Illness*. New York: Simon & Schuster, 1992.

Boenisch, Ed and C. Michele Haney. *The Stress Owner's Manual*. San Luis Obispo, Calif.: Impact Publishers, 1996.

Buscaglia, L. *Living, Loving, and Learning*. New York: Fawcett Books, 1982.

Butler, G. and T. Hope. *Managing Your Mind*. New York: Oxford University Press, 1995.

Cousins, N. *Anatomy of an Illness*. New York: W. W. Norton & Company, Inc., 1979.

Donovan, B. M. "Imagery: Awakening the Inner Healer." In *Holistic Nursing: A Handbook for Practice*. B. M. Dossey, L. Keagan, C. E. Guzzetta, and L. G. Kolkmeier, eds. Rockville, Md.: Aspen, 1988.

Eliot, Robert. *From Stress to Strength*. New York: Bantam Books, 1994.

———. "Relationship of Emotional Stress to the Heart." *Heart Disease and Stroke* 2 no. 3: 243–46 (1993).

Frankl, V. *Man's Search for Meaning*. 3rd ed. New York: Pocket Books, 1984.

Ganster, D. C. and B. Victor. "The Impact of Social Support on Mental and Physical Health." *British Journal of Medical Psychology* 61: 3–17 (1988).

Hodgkinson, L. *Smile Therapy: How Smiling and Laughter Can Change Your Life*. London: Optima, 1987.

Larkin, D. M. "Therapeutic Suggestion." *Relaxation and Imagery: Tools for Therapeutic Communication and Intervention*. P. R. Zahourek, ed. Philadelphia: W.B. Saunders, 1988.

McKay, M. *Self-Esteem*. Oakland, Calif.: New Harbinger Publications, 1987.

Munro, B. H., A. M. Creamer, M. R. Haggerty, and F. S. Cooper. "Effect of Relaxation Therapy of Post-Myocardial Infarction Patients' Rehabilitation." *Nursing Research* 37, no. 4: 231–35 (1988).

Payne, Rosemary. *Relaxation Techniques*. Edinburgh: Churchill Livingstone, 1995.

Peale, N. V. *The Power of Positive Thinking*. Englewood Cliffs, N.J.: Prentice-Hall, 1987.

*"Physical Activity and Cardiovascular Health."* NIH Consens Statement, 13(3): 1–33 (Dec. 18–20, 1995).

Schiraldi, Glenn. *Conquer Anxiety, Worry, and Nervous Fatigue: A Guide to a Greater Peace*. Ellicott City, Md.: Chevron Publishing Corporation, 1997.

Seaward, Brian Luke. *Managing Stress: Principles and Strategies for Health and Well-Being*. Boston: Jones and Barlett Publishers, 1994.

Seeman, T. E. and S. L. Syme. "Social Networks and Coronary Artery Disease: A Comparison of the Structure and Function of Social Relations as Predictors of Disease." *Psychosomatic Medicine* 49: 341–54 (1987).

Strecher, Victor, Gerard Seijts, Gerjo Kok, et al. "Goal Setting As a Strategy for Health Behavior Change." *Health Education Quarterly* 22: 190–200 (1995).

Van Dixhoorn, J., H. J. Duivenvorden, J. A. Stall, J. Pool, and F. Varghag. "Cardiac Events After Myocardial Infarction: Possible Effect of Relaxation Therapy." *European Heart Journal* 8: 1210–14 (1987).

Wallston, Barbara, Sheryle Alagna, Brenda McEvoy DeVellis, and Robert DeVellis. "Social Support and Physical Health." *Health Psychology* 2: 367–91 (1983).


CHAPTER SEVEN

American Heart Association World Wide Web Site. *Heart and Stroke Guide Section*, 1996.

Armstrong, L. E. and J. E. Dziados. "Effects of Heat Exposure on the Exercising Adult." *Sports Physical Therapy*. D. B. Bernhardt, ed. New York: Churchill Livingstone, 1986.

Atkin, Charles and Lawrence Wallack, eds. *Mass Communication and Public Health*. Newbury Park, Calif.: Sage Publications, 1990.

Authority of U.S. Pharmacopedia. *The Guide to Heart Medicines*. New York: Avon Books, 1996.

Carter, J. E. and C. V. Gisolfi. "Fluid Replacement During and After Exercise in the Heat." *Medicine and Science in Sports and Exercise* 21: 532 (1989).

Claremont, A. D. "Taking Winter in Stride Requires Proper Attire." *The Physician and Sports Medicine* 4: 65 (1976).

Committee for the Study of the Future of Public Health Division of Health Care Services Institute of Medicine. *The Future of Public Health*. Washington, D.C.: National Academy Press, 1988.

Covello, Vincent, Detlog von Winterfeldt, and Paul Slovic. "Communicating Scientific Information About Health and Environmental Risks: Problems and Opportunities from a Social and Behavioral Perspective." *Uncertainties in Risk Assessment and Risk Management*. V. Covello, A. Moghisi, and V. R. R. Uppuluri, eds. New York: Plenum Press, 1986.

"Dealing with Your Doctor." *Women's Health Watch* 10, no. 1 (January 1994).

"Facts About Air Pollution and Exercise" (pamphlet). American Lung Association, 1990.

Frishman, R. "Don't Be a Wimp in the Doctor's Office." *The Harvard Health Letter* 21: 1–2 (August 1996).

Handal, Kathleen. *The American Red Cross First Aid and Safety Book.* Boston: Little, Brown and Company, 1992.

Juneau, M., M. Johnstone, L. Lariee, et al. "Effect of Cold Upon Ischemic Threshold in Patients with Stable Angina, Magnitude and Mechanism." *Journal of American Cardiology* 13: 184A (1989).

Leathar, D. S., G. B. Hastings, and J. K. Davies, eds. *Health Education and the Media.* Oxford: Pergamon Press, 1981.

McArdle, William, Frank Katch, and Victor Katch. *Exercise Physiology: Energy, Nutrition, and Human Performance.* 4th ed. Baltimore, Md.: Williams & Wilkins, 1996.

Metropolitan Washington Council on Governments. "Air Quality Forecast and Action Guide." Washington, D.C.

Vogel, J. A., B. H. Jones, and P. B. Rock. "Environmental Considerations in Exercise Testing and Training." *Resource Manual for Guidelines for Exercise Testing and Prescription.* Steven Blair, Patricia Painter, Russell Pate, L. Kent Smith, and C. Barr Taylor, eds. Philadelphia: Lea and Febiger, 1988.

## CHAPTER EIGHT

Prochaska, James and Carlo DiClemente. "Transtheoretical Therapy: Toward a More Integrative Model of Change." *Psychotherapy: Theory, Research, and Practice* 51: 161–73 (1982).

Prochaska, James, Carlo DiClemente, and John Norcross. "In Search of How People Change." *American Psychologist* 47: 1102–114 (1992).

Strecher, Victor, Brenda McEvoy DeVellis, Marshall Becker, and Irwin Rosenstock. "The Role of Self-Efficacy in Achieving Health Behavior Change." *Health Education Quarterly* 13: 73–91 (1986).

Strecher, Victor, Gerard Seijts, Gerjo Kok, et al. "Goal Setting as a Strategy for Health Behavior Change." *Health Education Quarterly* 22: 190–200 (1995).

# INDEX

❦